Digital Democracy

The exponential growth of new Information and Communication Technologies (ICTs) such as the Internet, alongside growing concerns about the failure of advanced societies to live up to the democratic idea, has produced much interest in the prospects for a 'digital democracy'.

On one side, evangelists of the emancipatory potential of ICTs describe the emergence of an electronic social commons in which citizens can deliberate in an informed manner on matters of collective concern. However, on the other side there are those who present a vision of the death of democracy and the emergence of a 'Big Brother' state based upon electronic surveillance of citizens. By drawing together empirical evidence from Europe, the US and Canada, *Digital Democracy* attempts to separate the rhetoric from the reality concerning the actual and potential impacts of ICTs on democratic institutions and practice.

Digital Democracy considers how technological developments might combine with underlying social, economic and political conditions to produce new vehicles for democratic practice. It will provide invaluable reading for those studying social policy, politics and sociology, as well as for policy analysts, social scientists and computer scientists.

Barry N. Hague is Research Co-ordinator of the Community Informatics Research and Applications Unit (CIRA) based at the University of Teesside. **Brian D. Loader** is Co-director of CIRA and editor of the international journal *Information, Communication and Society* (Routledge), *The Governance of Cyberspace* (Routledge, 1997) and *The Cyberspace Divide* (Routledge, 1998).

Digital Democracy
Discourse and Decision Making
in the Information Age

**Edited by Barry N. Hague and
Brian D. Loader**

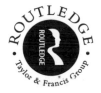

London and New York

First published 1999 by Routledge
11 New Fetter Lane, London EC4P 4EE

Simultaneously published in the USA and Canada
by Routledge
29 West 35th Street, New York, NY 10001

Routledge is an imprint of the Taylor & Francis Group

Typeset in Sabon by
The Florence Group, Stoodleigh, Devon
Printed and bound in Great Britain by
MPG Books Ltd, Bodmin

British Library Cataloguing in Publication Data
A catalogue record for this book is available from
the British Library

Library of Congress Cataloging in Publication Data
Digital democracy: discourse and decision making in the
Information Age/edited by Barry N. Hague and Brian D. Loader.
p. cm.
Chiefly based on papers presented at a conference sponsored
by the Community Informatics Research and Applications unit,
University of Teesside, UK.
Includes bibliographical references and index.
ISBN 0-415-19737-6 (hbk.).—ISBN 0-415-19738-4 (pbk.)
1. Public administration—Data processing—Congresses.
2. Administrative agencies—Data processing—Congresses.
3. Information technology—Political aspects—Congresses.
I. Hague, Barry N., 1961– II. Loader, Brian, 1958–.
JF1525.A8D54 1999
351'.0285–dc21   98–32052
                                                    CIP

ISBN 0-415-19737-6 (hbk)
ISBN 0-415-19738-4 (pbk)

Contents

Illustrations

Figures

Tables

Contributors

G. Scott Aikens is currently a Research Associate at Cambridge University funded by an ESRC research grant. Additionally, Dr Aikens co-founded MN E-Democracy, is a founding member and Board Director of UK Citizens Online Democracy, and developed the online strategy for Nexus – the policy and ideas network.

Stephen Coleman is Director of Studies at The Hansard Society for Parliamentary Government. He has worked with the Parliamentary Office of Science and Technology on online discussion projects and was an adviser for the publication of their 1997 'Electronic Government' report. He is working on 'The Virtual Parliament' project; an extensive study of Government web sites; and a forthcoming book, *Interactive Media and Democratic Culture*.

Sharon Docter received her JD from the University of California, Los Angeles and her PhD from the Annenberg School for Communication, University of Southern California. She currently serves as the Chair of the Communication Department at California Lutheran University in Thousand Oaks, California, and is the North American Book Review Editor of *Information, Communication and Society* (Routledge). Her research concerns the way in which the First Amendment may be applied to the regulation of new communication technology, as well as the degree to which First Amendment considerations have shaped the design of new technologies and policy governing use.

William H. Dutton is Professor of Communication in the Annenberg School for Communication at the University of Southern California, where he directs the Communication Management Program. From 1993–96, Professor Dutton was National Director of the UK's Programme on Information and Communication

Technologies (PICT), while a Visiting Professor at Brunel University, where he was also a Fulbright Scholar in 1986–87. His most recent book is *Society on the Line: Information Politics in the Digital Age* (Oxford University Press, 1999).

Barry N. Hague is a Senior Lecturer in Social Policy, and Research Coordinator for the Community Informatics Research and Applications Unit (CIRA), at the University of Teesside. He is reviews editor for the international journal *Information, Communication and Society* (Routledge) and has research interests in community informatics and organisation theory.

Matthew Hale is a second year doctoral candidate in Public Administration at the University of Southern California. He received his BA in Political Science at the University of California at Irvine and his MPA from USC. His research interests include technology and media effects in the political and governance process.

Hans Johansson lectures in Political Science at Mid-Sweden University. His main research areas are ICTs in politics and higher education in Sweden.

Klaus Lenk is Professor of Public Administration at the University of Oldenburg, Germany. His research interests include administrative policy and reform, information technology and its impact upon public administration, organisational forms and ICTs, the political implications of ICTs, and the information polity (regulatory issues, public access, data protection, infrastructures of information provision). He has published extensively on all of these issues.

Brian D. Loader is Co-Director of the Community Informatics Research and Applications Unit (CIRA) based at the University of Teesside. He edits the international journal *Information, Communication and Society* (iCS) published by Routledge. He is joint-editor of *Towards a Post-Fordist Welfare State?* (Routledge, 1994) and is editor of *The Governance of Cyberspace* (Routledge, 1997) and *The Cyberspace Divide* (Routledge, 1998).

Trevor Locke gained his Masters Degree in Urban Policy Studies from Leicester Polytechnic (now De Montfort University). He runs a locality web site for the Blaby area of Leicestershire which features several areas devoted to local politics. He works as an internet consultant for a Leicester computer company and maintains a large number of web sites which he has constructed for both public and private sector clients. He is a member of the Leicestershire, Leicester and Rutland Telematics Strategy Forum.

Anna Malina is an Associate Lecturer in Visual Communication and a doctoral researcher attached to the Communications and Information Studies Department at Queen Margaret College in Edinburgh. She has research interests in community informatics, particularly the social shaping of community-based electronic networks. Her current research critically examines the background, emergence, development, use, significance and ramifications of the Craigmillar Community Information Service (CCIS), a community-based electronic network situated in Craigmillar, Edinburgh.

Eileen Milner is Principal Lecturer in Information Management in the School of Law, Governance and Information Management at the University of North London. She leads research in the closely aligned areas of information and knowledge management in the public sector. She has undertaken considerable research activity in North America and Australia on the development of information and knowledge strategies and is currently working on *Managing Information and Knowledge in the Public Sector*, a book to be published by Routledge late in 1999.

Richard K. Moore worked for 30 years in the computer software industry, doing research and development for such Silicon Valley firms as Xerox PARC, Apple Computer and Oracle. For the past four years he has been a resident of Ireland where he has been writing on the topics of globalisation, corporate power and political activism. He has presented several papers at academic conferences and was invited to speak at the UN in Geneva on the history and future directions of the World Trade Organization. He is currently developing a book, *Globalization and the Revolutionary Imperative*, which can be found on his web site at: http://cyberjournal.org.

Juliet Musso has a doctorate in Public Policy from University of California Berkeley, and is an assistant professor at University of Southern California. Her research has focused on the effects of federalism institutions on service delivery and political 'voice' and 'exit'. She is currently researching the effects of internet technology, and of neighbourhood council structures, on local democratic participation.

Paul Nixon is a Senior Lecturer in Comparative Social Policy, and European Project Co-ordinator for CIRA, at the University of Teesside. He is presently Visiting Professor of European Integration at Mid-Sweden University. His most recent publications are as follows: 'Football and fanzines: observations on the English experience', in J. Dragowski, D. Knauf and I. Watson (eds) *Alive and Kicking: Fussball zwischen Deutschland und England*, Berlin: Argument Verlag, 1995; 'Watching the World Cup watchers', *NewLeaf* No 3. Summer 1996; and 'A never closer union: Malcolm Bradbury's The Gravy Train Goes East', in S. Fendler and R. Wittlinger (eds) *The Idea of Europe in Literature* forthcoming.

Elisabeth Richard, Director, Corporate and Public Affairs, Canadian Policy Research Networks, is responsible for strategies to communicate results of research and to help build relationships with policy makers, funders, opinion leaders and the public. Elisabeth created the Government of Canada Primary Internet Site, based on a strategy of timeliness, community participation and responsiveness. She co-authored the G7 White Paper on Governments OnLine and Democracy, and managed the Web Publishing services at Government Telecommunications and Informatics Services. Previously a broadcaster and journalist with the Canadian Broadcasting Corporation and Radio-Canada, Elisabeth graduated from the Economics and Finance program of the Institut d'Etudes Politiques de Paris.

Christopher Weare is an Assistant Professor at the University of Southern California where he has taught since 1994. Prior to receiving his PhD, Professor Weare received a BA *cum laude* from Harvard in 1983 and an MPP from Berkeley in 1987. Professor Weare has published widely in the areas of public policy, telecommunications regulation, and the use of technology by local governments.

C. William R. Webster is a researcher at the Centre for the Study of Telematics and Governance (CSTAG), Glasgow Caledonian University. He is currently completing a doctorate on the policy processes surrounding the uptake of Closed Circuit Television (CCTV) surveillance cameras in public places across the UK, and has a number of publications in the area. His other research interests include developments in the delivery of electronic public services and citizenship, governance in the Information Age, electronic democracy and the relevance of telecommunications policy and regulation to these innovations. William is a member of the European Group of Public Administration (EGPA) Permanent Study Group on 'Informatization in Public Administration' and the European Union Co-operation in the Field of Science and Technological Research (COST) Action 14 'Government and Democracy in the Information Age' (GaDIA) research programme.

Anthony G. Wilhelm is Program Director of Communications Policy and Practice (CPP) at the Benton Foundation, an organization working to realize the social benefits made possible by the public interest use of communications. CPP promotes public interest values and noncommercial services for the evolving information society through research, policy analysis, print and online publishing.

Preface

The focus for this book is a critical exploration of the potential for new information and communications technologies (ICTs), such as the internet, to contribute to 'strong democracy' based around citizen-to-citizen deliberation and strengthened links between governments and the governed. The book is premised on the belief that an understanding of the dialectical relationship between technology and society is essential to a critical understanding of 'digital democracy' initiatives. Further, the majority of the book's contributors lend weight to the argument that, if ICTs are to play a significant role in the achievement of strong democracy, then they must be grounded in community networks. Finally, this volume, by drawing upon empirical evidence from a number of countries, seeks to contribute to the separation of the rhetoric from the reality concerning experiments in, and prospects for, digital democracy.

These concerns formed the basis for a conference organised by the Community Informatics Research and Applications Unit (CIRA) based at the University of Teesside, from which the majority of chapters in this volume originate. All the chapters have been substantially reviewed in the light of the lively and productive debate during the conference, and additional contributions have been sought to enhance that debate further.

We would like to take this opportunity to thank the participants in the original conference for their contributions to what was a stimulating and enjoyable event. The fact that it was so enjoyable was, in no small part, down to the professional way in which the event was organised by members of the CIRA team. Particular thanks are due in this regard to Jo Brudenell (who also has our deepest appreciation for her efforts in dealing with the administrative obstacles to pulling this collection together), June Ions and Paul Haslock.

Thanks are also due to the team at Routledge for their support and forbearance, in particular Commissioning Editor Heather Gibson and her colleague Fiona Bailey. Last, but not least, we would like to express our heartfelt gratitude to our partners Dorothy Hague and Kim Loader for their support and understanding and to our 4 year olds – Declan Hague, Christopher Loader and William Loader – for providing a sense of perspective.

Barry N. Hague and
Brian D. Loader

Part I

Digital democracy: concepts and issues

1 Digital democracy: an introduction

Barry N. Hague and
Brian D. Loader

There exists a growing body of thought that articulates the belief that recent developments in information and communications technologies (ICTs) contain within them the potential to facilitate 'quantum leaps in the field of democratic politics' (Becker 1998: 343). For Becker, these amount to no less than a paradigm shift in the process of the understanding of democratic governance.

A variety of models, experiments and initiatives are emerging in response to the challenge of (re)invigorating democratic institutions and practice by utilising ICTs. These initiatives are variously grouped in the literature under the umbrella of 'electronic democracy', 'tele-democracy' and 'cyberdemocracy'. The term 'digital democracy' is preferred here since it is the bringing together of existing electronic technologies through developments in digital data transfer that unleashes the potential of ICTs.[1] At present, the notion of digital democracy can refer to a fairly wide range of technological applications including televised 'people's parliaments' or citizens' juries, e-mail access to electronic discussion groups, and public information kiosks (DEMOS 1997). It is not the aim of this collection to provide a comprehensive coverage of such initiatives; this task is left to other authors. Neither is it intended to provide detailed accounts of competing models of democracy, their relative merits and the underlying conditions required for their realisation (see Held 1987). Still less is the collection intended to join arms with either the cyber-libertarian vision of a digital utopia (Barlow 1996) or the technophobic distopian nightmares of a surveillance society (Davies 1996). Both of these scenarios lean too much towards technological determinism. It is important to recognise that new ICT applications, whether directed at enhancing democracy or not, emerge out of the 'dialectical interaction between technology and society' (Castells 1997: 5); they are subject to 'social shaping' (Kubicek *et al.* 1997) and, as such, they will be influenced by such factors as technological precedent, culture (political or otherwise), legal frameworks, etc., and will emerge through the activities of human agents, constrained as they are by existing power relations.

The aims of this book, then, are as follows. First, to address the question of what a 'strong democracy' based on extensive use of ICTs might look like. Second, to explore the likely effects of alternative underlying social, economic and political conditions on the 'digital democracy' we actually achieve. Third, to draw together international case study material with a view to separating the rhetoric from the reality concerning the current impacts of ICTs on democratic practice. Fourth, to draw lessons from this case study material concerning barriers to the realisation of 'digital democracy', the pursuit of alternative 'agendas', and the emergence of unintended consequences from the application of ICTs. Before elaborating upon these aims, let us briefly rehearse the justifications for such a project.

Digital democracy: why the interest?

The major justifications for (re)visiting democratic practice in the light of an emergent Information Age are twofold. The first concerns a growing perception that current political institutions, actors and practice in advanced liberal democracies are in a frail condition and are held in poor public regard. The second concerns a belief that the current period of rapid social, economic and political change, which may signal an emergent Information Age, provides opportunities hitherto unavailable to rethink and, if necessary, radically overhaul or replace those institutions, actors and practice.

Representative models of democracy have come to characterise many twentieth-century societies. It is only by conceding a great deal of their power, runs the argument, to a smaller number of politicians whose job it is to represent their common interests that citizens can live in a democratic society at all. Conversely, its opponents have argued that elected representatives often do not represent the 'will of the people' and are prone to elitism (Mitchels 1962). More recently, politicians have become tarnished with allegations of sleaze, corruption, self-seeking behaviour and sound-bite politics that may have produced widespread disillusionment and apathy amongst citizens and particularly the young (Wilkinson and Mulgan 1995). It is against this background that we have to assess where the notion of digital democracy fits in.

The second reason why a focus on 'digital democracy' is appo-site concerns the notion that society is undergoing a paradigmatic shift. Castells quotes palaeontologist Stephen J. Gould thus:

> The history of life, as I read it, is a series of stable states, punc-tuated at rare intervals by major events that occur with great rapidity and help to establish the next stable era ... [A]t the end of the twentieth century, we are living through one of these rare intervals in history. An interval characterised by trans-formation of our 'material culture' by the works of a new technological paradigm organised around information techno-logies.
>
> (Castells 1997: 29)

It is the assumption here that such an interval may indeed be in progress and, furthermore, that it is during such periods of upheaval that the potential for human agency in the shaping of our collec-tive future is at its greatest (cf. Hoggett 1990). It is for this reason that deliberation on the likely and desired future shape of our polit-ical institutions and practice, and the potential role of ICTs therein, is paramount. Contributions to the debate are to be sought from and between various academic disciplines and fields (including polit-ical science, sociology, public administration, economics, law, information management and computer science) as well as from public servants, ICT professionals and lay enthusiasts, and the wider citizenry. It is hoped that this edited collection makes an important, if modest, contribution to this end.

A vision of 'strong democracy'

There are already a number of competing conceptions of democracy, and it is not entirely clear whether electronic democracy is being put forward as a different variant. Typically, debate in recent years has tended to focus upon a kind of continuum, with participatory democracy (Pateman 1970) at one end of the scale and representa-tive democratic models at the other. Participatory democracy has been seen to be the closest approximation to direct democracy, with its exhortation to involve the public in decision-making pro-cesses. Its critics have pointed out that examples of such participatory behaviour tend to be rather limited to a few instances of local poli-tics and workplace groups. Furthermore, its advocates have often paid less attention to those who do not wish constantly to embrace political debate and action. Moreover, the size and complexity of modern nation-states has meant that the citizen has little realistic opportunity (or perhaps desire) to influence their environment beyond the village pump.

Is there something qualitatively different about digital democracy that gives it a new conceptual status? As we have seen, at present the notion of digital democracy is used to refer to a range of technological applications and experiments. Whilst such experiments are useful for improving existing representative democratic institutions, and the huge increase in local, regional and state government web-sites should be welcomed as attempts to improve the citizen–government interface, they do not seem to us to constitute an entirely new democratic system. As is frequently the case, ICTs are often used to augment existing practice rather than revolutionise institutions.

It is assumed here, however, that the evangelists of the internet have something more in mind when they extol the virtues of digital democracy, which suggests that power will transfer to the *demos* once they are armed with ICTs. In its extreme form, the internet is conceived as an electronic forum comprising a vast network of liberated and equal citizens of the world capable of debating all facets of their existence without fear of control from national sovereign authorities (Barlow 1996). The limitations of this cyber-libertarian approach have been dealt with elsewhere (Loader 1997). It is worth reminding ourselves, however, of the key features of interactive media that are claimed to offer the potential for the development of a new variety of democracy:

- Interactivity – users may communicate on a many-to-many reciprocal basis.
- Global network – communication is not fettered by nation-state boundaries.
- Free speech – net users may express their opinions with limited state censorship.
- Free association – net users may join virtual communities of common interest.
- Construction and dissemination of information – net users may produce and share information that is not subject to official review or sanction.
- Challenge to professional and official perspectives – state and professional information may be challenged.
- Breakdown of nation-state identity – users may begin to adopt global and local identities.

Whilst all of these features raise important questions for empirical study and debate, their existence seems somewhat restricted at the present time. Welcome though existing initiatives are, democracy is about more than voting or providing better public information to the citizen: electronic plebiscites and public information kiosks are simply not sufficient conditions to affirm the existence of digital democracy. Democracy has at its heart self-determination, participation, voice and autonomy. It is a political culture that includes a wide range of realms for self-development and mutual collective expression.

If an enhanced form of digital democracy is to emerge, it would seem reasonable to speculate, on the basis of the foregoing discussion, that it is likely to be a hybrid democratic model containing elements of both participatory and representative forms of democracy. The concept of 'democratic autonomy' developed by David Held (1996) is useful in developing this line of argument. Held's model, like the argument presented in this chapter, is predicated upon an inclusive definition of politics:

> politics is a phenomenon found in and between all groups, institutions and societies, cutting across public and private life. It is expressed in all the activities of co-operation, negotiation and struggle over the use and distribution of resources. It is involved in all the relations, institutions and structures which are implicated in the activities of production and reproduction in the life of societies.
>
> (Held 1996: 310)

If we accept this inclusive definition of politics, then 'strong democracy' must offer the opportunity for the 'participation of citizens in all those decisions concerning issues which impinge upon and are important to them (i.e. us)' (ibid.). The practical achievement of such a state must involve a symbiotic relationship between both representative and participatory democratic forms and, for Held, requires that democracy be 'reconceived as a double-sided phenomenon: concerned on the one hand, with the *re*-form of state power and, on the other hand, with the restructuring of civil society' (ibid.: 316).

Held's 'principle of autonomy' requires the protection of individual rights and, hence, makes some form of constitutional government, overseen by elected representatives, necessary. The challenge is to reform such government so as to circumscribe its power to impinge upon individual autonomy whilst retaining the authority to uphold it, and to make its business accountable to all citizens. At the same time, the 'principle of autonomy' requires that '[people] should be able to participate in a process of debate and deliberation, open to all on a free and equal basis, about matters of pressing public concern' (ibid.: 302).

From the foregoing discussion, certain questions, which are open to empirical investigation, begin to emerge in relation to the role of ICTs in the creation of 'strong democracy':

- To what extent might ICTs facilitate more accountable government (national and local)?
- To what extent might ICTs be used to create a more informed (about the business of government) citizenry?
- To what extent might ICTs facilitate citizen participation in decision making concerning affairs of state?
- To what extent might ICTs facilitate participation by citizens in 'debate and deliberation', on a 'free and equal basis', concerning affairs of state?
- To what extent might ICTs facilitate participation by citizens in 'debate and deliberation', on a 'free and equal basis', within civil society?
- To what extent might ICTs facilitate citizen participation, on a 'free and equal basis', in collective decision making concerning issues that impinge upon them within civil society?

Each of the contributors to this book addresses one or more of the above questions. The chapters in Part II are concerned primarily with developments relating to the democratisation of the state. Those in Part III focus upon developments in civil society. A common theme for each of the chapters is a concern with the potential for ICTs, often but not exclusively focused upon the interactive characteristics of the internet, to foster more deliberative, discursive, democratic forms. This reflects, we feel, a mutual recognition of the centrality of what Robert Putnam (1993a) calls 'social capital', which promotes civic engagement and interaction between citizens concerning matters of common concern – to any notion of 'strong democracy'.

Two further themes that emerge throughout the book, and which are central to the prospects for 'strong democracy', are those concerning access to and ownership and control of those ICTs holding potential for democratic reform, and it is to these that we now turn.

The question of access

Consideration of the potential of ICTs to facilitate the creation of 'strong democracy' inevitably raises concerns over access. Typically, such concerns, particularly as expressed by governments, have focused on broadening access to ICT hardware and software and providing widely available basic training in their use (the British government-sponsored 'IT for All' and 'Computers Don't Bite' initiatives provide good examples). As important and welcome as these considerations and the initiatives that flow from them are, we feel that the question of access raises a range of issues that move beyond a concern with physical access to ICTs

Access to ICTs

Naturally, the question of who has access to the latest ICTs, and who does not, is an important one. The potential of ICTs to facilitate 'strong democracy' must be seriously questioned if people are systematically denied access on the basis of economic status, gender, geographic location, educational attainment, and so on. Advocates of the emancipatory potential of the internet, for example, would do well to remember that it remains the domain of a relatively elite association of mainly white, male, professional people from advanced societies (Holderness 1998). Of course, it might be argued that the exponential growth of connectivity means that the unconnected 'information poor' will become an increasingly small group that can be targeted and prioritised through state-sponsored initiatives. This would, however, be somewhat to miss the point. It is highly likely that the achievement of mass connectivity will coincide with the creation of a commercially dominated (and owned?) 'global digital high-bandwidth network'. By the time such a network is in place, the technological paradigm that will both constrain the types of activity and interactivity that are possible in cyberspace and, more fundamentally, provide the conceptual tools with which we seek to understand and shape cyberspace, may already be entrenched. Traffic around this network may bear little resemblance to the anarchic, global commons so beloved of internet enthusiasts today (see Chapter 3). As Castells states with his usual perceptiveness, 'while governments and futurologists speak of wiring classrooms, doing surgery at a distance and tele-consulting the Encyclopaedia Britannica, most of the actual construction of the new system focuses on "video-on-demand", tele-gambling and VR theme parks' (1997: 366).

Accepting our previous argument that the potential for human agency in the shaping of tomorrow's technologies is at present relatively strong, it becomes of paramount importance, to anyone genuinely concerned with 'strong democracy', that all citizens are exposed to the current capabilities of ICTs and are encouraged to consider whether and how they might be utilised to the betterment of their individual and collective lives. This is where state-sponsored initiatives to broaden access, like those mentioned earlier, can be found wanting. Such initiatives have been conceived and implemented in a very 'top down' manner. The underlying logic would appear to run along the following lines: ICTs are a good thing *per se*; those who can access and have the skills to utilise these ICTs will gain obvious advantages (primarily economic) for themselves and will be more useful (primarily economically) to society; better drag as many people as possible along to their nearest training provider, overcome their groundless fears and equip them with some basic computing skills. What is missing here is any attempt to ground awareness raising and training regarding ICTs in the everyday experience of individuals and communities and to allow them to decide for themselves what use ICTs may be to them.

It is this latter concern that underpins our work with CIRA (Community Informatics Research and Applications Unit) at the University of Teesside. It is our belief that the achievement of 'strong democracy' may be fundamentally dependent upon embedding ICTs within community networks and, at the same time, fostering remote connectivity. Market forces alone, however, are unlikely to ensure the necessary awareness, access and education for any but the most privileged members of advanced societies without financial inducement and regulation (Loader 1998). Furthermore, it may be too much to expect politicians and professionals to cede power to people through facilitating electronic interactivity. It must be remembered that much community empowerment frequently manifests itself as community action against the local and nation-state.

The extent to which the appropriate social and economic conditions may emerge to foster the development of 'strong democracy' may depend upon a negotiated outcome between service providers and communications industries, politicians and the action of communities themselves. Community Informatics, which is concerned with the study of the effects of ICTs on community development, restructuring and the confluence of social networks and electronic networks, is still too much in its infancy to cast much light on these still embryonic developments. Nonetheless, a number of communities in the USA and Europe are experimenting with the development of their own information systems which may act as early pointers to future developments.[2]

Some may argue that much of the use being made of ICTs within local communities has little bearing on the goals of (re)engaging people in politics and strengthening the democratic process. Such an argument is, however, inextricably linked to the notion that politics is 'what governments do'. Taking the inclusive definition of politics adopted earlier, any and all community use of ICTs to enhance self-determination and promote collective endeavour is central to the achievement of 'strong democracy'.

Access to information

Providing physical access to ICTs is one thing; giving citizens good reason to want to make use of them is quite another. This requires that we move away from Information Age rhetoric about the value of ICTs *per se*, and scare tactics concerning the social and economic exclusion awaiting individuals and communities that do not 'get wired'. To risk stating the obvious, the value of ICTs to citizens is heavily contingent upon the type and quality of 'content' to which they provide access. If ICTs are to promote 'strong democracy', then attention must be paid to providing relevant information, in a user-friendly format, at times, in locations and at a cost that do not present barriers to access. Following the approach to Community Informatics that is advocated here, the initial focus of such attention should not be upon ICTs but rather upon existing information needs, patterns of information retrieval, and barriers to accessing information. From here, communities themselves can be involved in considering how ICTs might be applied to meet their information needs (which may, quite legitimately, range from accessing news about the local football team to finding out about current government policy proposals). Furthermore, armed with knowledge concerning the potential of ICTs to meet their information needs, communities are empowered to apply pressure on the relevant information providers (across public, private and voluntary sectors) if the required information is not forthcoming. Perhaps the most exciting development of all, however, is that the 'many-to-many' nature of communications facilitated by the latest ICTs, means that citizens and communities can become information providers themselves, sharing information about themselves and shaping an identity for dissemination within the local community and beyond to the wired world.

Access to community networks

The concept of community, whilst still widely used in common parlance, has lost favour within academic circles due to the imprecise use of the term (Plant *et al.* 1980). The difficulty with notions of community is that they tend to focus on internal relationships within a defined locality without reference to ties and links outside the geographical domain (Crow and Allan 1994: 177). Traditional studies have overemphasised local cohesion and solidarity and 'as a result they failed to recognise or address properly the difference and varied levels of commitment and exchange which most people sustain within their networks' (ibid.: 181–2). In more recent years, however, 'network analysis' has offered the prospect of tackling the problem of boundary definition by considering communities as networks of individuals connected both locally and remotely (Wellman and Berkowitz 1988; Scott 1991).

Such a focus on community networks allows the exploration of how ICTs might foster widened and deepened interaction between and within communities (whether geographic communities or communities of interest). The network metaphor that underpins Information Age technologies can be extended to encompass the co-ordination of social life, allowing exploration of the attributes that underpin and sustain social networks, such as *solidarity, altruism, loyalty, reciprocity* and *trust* (Thompson 1993), and the extent to which electronic networks might help to maintain, strengthen and proliferate such ties. In short, it allows an exploration of the role of ICTs in building 'social capital'.

The above is not intended to place the current authors alongside those virtual communitarians (see e.g. Rheingold 1993) who herald the arrival of a freely accessible electronic 'social commons'. Electronic community networks will overlie, but potentially enhance and expand, existing social networks and, as such, will be subject to the same economic and political constraints. It is highly probable, and open to empirical test, that those who are well networked in 'real space' will be those who are well networked in cyberspace and vice versa. Despite this, and perhaps because of it, disseminating the ability to network electronically as widely as possible must be central to the creation of a 'strong democracy' facilitated by ICTs.

Access to decision makers

A common criticism of advanced liberal democracies is that governments have become isolated from and unresponsive to the citizens on whose behalf they ostensibly act (see Chapter 8). 'Strong democracy' requires strong and interactive links between the state and civil society, between government and the governed. Much of the rhetoric about the potential for digital democracy, and much existing practice, centres on the ability of interactive ICTs to overcome barriers of time and space and facilitate both the flow of information from governments to citizens and direct citizen 'feedback' and participation in the business of government. So we have the prospect of national and local governments interacting with citizens via web sites, e-mail addresses and public information kiosks. We also have experiments with electronic voting, electronic voter guides, citizen juries and the like. However, it must be said that, on the evidence of contributions to this volume (see Part II), practical initiatives to date have largely failed to live up to the rhetoric. The evidence would suggest that government-sponsored initiatives display three common traits: first, a greater willingness to utilise ICTs to put out information to citizens than to use them as a vehicle for citizen feedback and participation; second, a tendency to focus on providing public service information to 'users' or 'customers', as opposed to outlining information and justifying policies for 'citizens'; and third, in the rare cases where input from the public is sought, a tendency to seek aggregate 'consumer/citizen' views (via e.g. electronic opinion polling, referenda, etc.) on predetermined issues rather than to encourage discourse and deliberation amongst citizens and allow an input to agenda setting. Of course, there is nothing about ICTs *per se* that encourages such traits: they are the product of social shaping. What 'strong democracy' requires is government committed to open and meaningful dialogue with the citizenry. What we should not expect is that the push towards such a condition will come from governments themselves.

Access to a basic source of income

It would be wrong to leave our consideration of the questions of access, which must be addressed and resolved before the vision of a 'strong democracy' facilitated by ICTs might be realised, without exposing the hype surrounding digital democracy to some sobering economic and political realities. The extensive use of ICTs to facilitate dialogue and deliberation amongst and between citizens and government, even if 'access' is ostensibly open to all, will never be sufficient on its own to foster a 'strong democracy' in which all citizens can, in practice, participate. That requires a more fundamental economic restructuring to provide all citizens with a minimum economic resource base; as Galbraith boldly put it:

> there is, first, the absolute, inescapable requirement that everyone in the good ... society has a basic source of income. And if this is not available from the market system ... it must come from the state. Nothing, let us not forget, sets a stronger limit on the liberty of the citizen than a total absence of money (1994, p. 2).
>
> (Held 1996: 319)

In considering the emancipatory potential of ICTs, we should never lose sight of such realities.

What the above also highlights is the central importance of issues relating to ownership and control of ICTs. The contribution that ICTs might make to the achievement of 'strong democracy' will be largely dependent on the overriding objectives of those who control the design, application and use of new systems.

Ownership and control

We have already described the form of multimedia system that may become commonplace through cable company and satellite distribution (i.e. one based on 'video-on-demand, tele-gambling and VR theme parks' [Castells 1997: 366]). Such a system offers little scope for interactive democratic expression. Instead, it offers a picture of a network with predefined structures of debate and very little opportunity for the use and development of alternative discourse. Whilst this form of electronic democracy may be appealing to a new breed of politicians such as Ross Perot, Bill Clinton and Tony Blair as a means of connecting directly with the people, it is also susceptible to manipulation and requires little active participation. As Castells remarks, 'who are the *interacting* and who are the *interacted* in the new system ... largely frames the system of domination and the processes of liberation in the informational society' (ibid.: 374).

The driving forces behind the development of what Castells calls the multimedia system are not governments but businesses. Indeed, the whole system may already be controlled by a very small number of global corporations (see Chapter 3). This also may have a significant impact upon the shaping of the media and its consequences for diversity and cultural difference:

The price to pay for inclusion in the system is to adapt to its logic, to its language, to its points of entry, to its encoding and decoding. This is why it is so critical for different kinds of social effects that there should be the development of a multinodal, horizontal network of communication, of internet type, instead of a centrally dispatched multimedia system, as in the video-on-demand configuration.

(Castells 1997: 374)

Left entirely to the commercial sector, a 'centrally dispatched multimedia system' is what is likely to emerge and, potentially, squeeze out the internet as currently configured (see Chapter 3). It is imperative, therefore, that governments take a more proactive stance than is currently apparent. For, as Castells suggests,

What must be retained for the understanding of the relationship between technology and society is that the role of the state, by either stalling, unleashing, or leading technological innovation, is a decisive factor in the overall process, as it expresses and organises the social and cultural forces that dominate in a given space and time.

(Castells 1997: 13)

Any optimism about the prospects for 'strong democracy' facilitated by ICTs must, then, be based on evidence that there is a will amongst governments to embrace the concept of 'strong democracy' and to be at the leading edge in developing and utilising ICT infrastructure and applications that might facilitate its achievement. The chapters in Part II provide interesting reading in this regard.

Of course, central to our argument in this introductory chapter has been the claim that, if ICTs are to play a significant role in the achievement of 'strong democracy', then the design and ownership of applications within civil society, at local community level, is also of vital importance. Specifically, we have argued that ICTs must be embedded within community networks that enjoy remote connectivity. After all, it may well be that in relation to the deployment of ICTs for democratic purposes, pressure from an active citizenry upon the state may be just as, if not more, important as pressure in the opposite direction. Let us not forget that community empowerment frequently manifests itself as action against the local and nation-state. The chapters in Part III are concerned with digital democracy initiatives within civil society.

Digital democracy: advancing the discourse

This collection is divided into three parts. The first, of which this introductory chapter forms a part, explores contrasting models of democracy and considers the extent to which ICTs can and may contribute to their realisation and enhancement. The second examines initiatives concerned with utilising ICTs to democratise the activities of the state. The third and final part focuses upon digital democracy initiatives within civil society.

Following the mapping of the terrain in this introductory chapter, Part I continues with Anna Malina's identification of key problems in relation to democracy and citizenship and consideration of strategies for emancipatory intervention to rejuvenate the public sphere. She argues that the prospects for 'electronic democratisation' will be dependent on whether 'information is packaged as an easily accessible "social good" or sold as a costly "consumer product" ', and that outcomes will be shaped by the typology of democracy practised and the perceptions of citizenship held. Picking up on one of the themes introduced in this chapter, Malina argues that ICTs will serve the cause of democratisation only if a prior will for strong democracy is established.

In a challenging polemic in Chapter 3, Richard Moore raises serious doubts over the prospect that the future cyberspace will be shaped by an overarching will for strong democracy. Arguing that the history of democracy is one of a 'see-saw' struggle between citizens at large and elite economic interests, he claims that the domination of cyberspace by a small number of vertically integrated transnational corporations, who conceive it primarily as a product distribution system and a means of opinion control, combined with the declining influence of nation-states brought about by the process of globalisation, will see the balance of power shift towards the economic elite. Under such circumstances, 'rather than the realisation of the democratic dream, cyberspace may turn out instead to be the ultimate Big Brother nightmare'. Moore's recommendations as to the actions necessary to mitigate against such a scenario revolve around the need for grass roots political activism, in effect amounting to a call for the (re)building of 'social capital'.

Part II opens with Eileen Milner's account of research on 'electronic government' undertaken at the University of North London (Chapter 4). Informed by the perspective provided by the disciplines of Information and Knowledge Management, this research has resulted in the development of an ideal type model for electronic government that is based upon a global review of practice. The model outlines a 'three-lane highway' to electronic government based around citizen involvement and satisfaction, employee involvement and satisfaction, and financial performance. Milner suggests that practice to date has been more characteristic of a 'single flow of traffic', with ICTs being seen as a tool to leverage bottom-line performance, the hard currency of which is cash savings. The results of this blinkered view, held by both politicians and senior public servants, are, she suggests, a waste of resources on a large scale and a missed opportunity to build a more positive interaction between government and the governed.

In a review of practice related to the Government of Canada Primary Internet Site, Elisabeth Richard, the site manager, provides a practitioner's perspective on the issues raised by attempts to utilise ICTs in pursuit of better governance (Chapter 5). She argues that currently a clear framework is lacking for the adaptation of traditional hierarchical public service structures to synergise with the new environment of links and nodes that comprises the Information Age. Amongst the issues she raises are the need for governments to develop techniques for 'mass listening' to complement the facility for 'mass talk' that characterises internet-related technologies; the need to consider how, when and by whom moderation of discourse between citizens and government should be applied; and the need to develop decision-making models that reflect a conceptualisation of the 'citizen as a partner'. Notwithstanding the problems and barriers identified, this chapter provides ample evidence of innovative and encouraging government practice.

With Klaus Lenk's contribution (Chapter 6), the focus shifts from national to local government. In providing a summary of ICT-supported information systems aimed at improving the quality of citizen participation in local planning, he demonstrates the potential of ICTs to facilitate citizen deliberation. For Lenk, the achievement of local democracy is a problem of organisation, and ICTs are, first and foremost, technologies of organisation: their value lies in their use to structure debates. He takes the view that the contribution that the unmoderated virtual marketplace of 'free-nets' can make to democratic discourse is limited. Where large numbers of people are concerned, and where issues are complex and policies overlap, there is a vital need to develop adequate procedures for structuring participatory decision-making processes.

Chapter 7 by Matthew Hale, Juliet Musso and Christopher Weare provides a detailed analysis of the content of some 290 Californian municipal web sites. Their analysis focuses on the extent to which such sites are used as a vehicle to address three major factors that inhibit citizen participation in the political system: inadequate civic education, citizen apathy, and a disconnection between citizens and their representatives. With some notable exceptions, they find that the potential for two-way communication through a web presence is not being fully realised. At the majority of sites they survey, 'information provision is patchy and the level of interactivity supported does not improve significantly on the telephone'. As regards more radical use of technology to foster citizen participation and deliberation, they find that current municipal use of web technology does little, if anything, to foster this type of democratic revitalisation.

Unlike the bulk of chapters in this book, William Webster's Chapter 8 is not concerned directly with the potential impacts of internet-related ICTs on democracy and the democratic process. Rather, he offers an analysis of the policy process leading to the widespread implementation of publicly funded CCTV systems. The significance of his contribution lies in the lessons to be learned about the motivations of government in relation to the utilisation of ICTs and about the manner in which government 'sells' the virtues of ICTs. Webster presents evidence that the policy process in relation to CCTV has been manipulated, through agenda setting and information shaping, to (re)assert societal control on the one hand and democratic renewal and legitimacy on the other. He argues that the case of CCTV provides evidence of the emergence of a more 'managed' form of democracy in which the 'packaging and marketing of public policy plays a central role in gaining support for those democratic institutions which represent citizens, make policy and deliver services'. Such a model of democracy is clearly far removed from that outlined in this introductory chapter and raises serious doubts as to the will of governments to achieve 'strong democracy'.

The final section of the volume is devoted to digital democracy initiatives in civil society. It opens with Paul Nixon and Hans Johansson's account in Chapter 9 of the use being made of ICTs by political parties in the case study countries of Sweden and Holland. They explore the impacts, actual and potential, of the increasing use of ICTs on party organisation and discipline, voting procedures and prospects for the development of a more discursive democracy. Nixon and Johansson contend that there is a continuing conflict within the political parties they studied between central control and local autonomy and that, whilst the Information Age presents opportunities for local democracy, these are often subsumed by the centralising tendencies of party machines. They also identify an imperative for political parties to reform their 'corporate vision' if they are to remain relevant in the Information Age, and postulate that the declining significance of the nation-state, coupled with the globalisation of information flows facilitated by internet-type technologies, may signify the advent of pan-European political representation on a scale far beyond the *ad hoc* voluntary collaborations witnessed thus far.

There is much rhetoric to suggest that the interactive fora of internet discussion lists and newsgroups provide an 'electronic agora' that supports citizen discourse and deliberation on matters political. In Chapter 10, Anthony Wilhelm seeks to separate the rhetoric from the reality by presenting a content analysis of a random sample of postings to Usenet newsgroups, self-identified as political, to ascertain the extent to which the interaction that takes place within them is consistent with the notion of 'democratic deliberation'. His findings are, on the whole, less than encouraging for those who champion the democratising influence of such forums. They are, he tells us, home to an array of overlapping, short-lived conversations, usually among like-minded individuals. Since sustained deliberation is rare within these newsgroups, they are, for Wilhelm, ineffective sounding boards for signalling and expounding issues and problems to be processed by government.

A far more positive spin on the potential for ICTs to create new deliberative mechanisms is presented by Scott Aikens in Chapter 11. Grounding his argument in the debate between John Dewey and Walter Lippman over the development of the American mass media, he presents evidence from three 'digital democracy' experiments with which he has had a personal involvement: Minnesota E-Democracy; UK Citizens Online Democracy (see also Chapter 12); and Nexus – the policy and ideas network. These experiments, Aikens claims, can usefully be described as 'Deweyan systems', intended to counter the 'dangerous tendencies of modern media politics' and 'support a new politics of individual freedom within cohesive communities'. For him, part of the potential for ICTs to promote democratic outcomes lies in their facilitation of 'multiple gateways to socialised intelligence', so that government by experts can be informed by 'community logics'. Picking up on one of the themes identified in this introductory chapter, Aikens further contends that, for this potential to be realised, experiments in digital democracy must be grounded in local communities, for it is here that social capital and political trust must be (re)established.

Stephen Coleman's Chapter 12 describes a further experiment in digital democracy, this time from Britain: UK Citizens Online Democracy (UKCOD). UKCOD was conceived as a politically neutral, online, democracy information and discussion service that allows citizens to interact freely with one another and with those elected to represent them. For Coleman, such experiments in digital democracy are 'not designed to replace representative democracy or to alter radically constitutionally established procedures of law making, parliamentary debate or scrutiny of the executive'. Rather, they aim to strengthen the 'deliberative input of the represented within a culture of democratic governance'. Coleman's chapter concludes with a useful attempt at identifying the principles that ought to underpin the future provision of electronic democracy services if such an aim is to be realised.

In Chapter 13, Trevor Locke provides an account of the development of community networks and the extent to which they can be used to overcome some of the barriers to the use of ICTs for democratic purposes by the citizenry at large. He expresses a belief, shared by many of the contributors to this book, that it is at the local level that the real potential for the use of ICTs to promote 'strong democracy' lies. He considers the concept of 'netactivism' – involving the use of the internet by citizens, geographic communities and communities of interest to organise and engage in political actions – and expresses optimism about the potential of people to 'en-personalise' the internet. Locke's optimism is not diminished by the observation that digital TV will quickly replace the internet as the infrastructure for the delivery of information. Indeed, he expresses the belief, by no means shared by all the book's contributors, that the interactivity and connectivity of the internet will find a 'much fuller life and vigour in the mass audiences of the TV set'.

Finally Sharon Docter and Bill Dutton's exposition of the social shaping of 'The Democracy Network' (DNet) in Chapter 14 reminds us of the importance of informing our analysis of digital democracy experiments with an understanding of the dialectical interaction between technology and society. DNet is an innovative electronic voter guide geared to the American electorate. Docter and Dutton chart how its overarching design was shaped by democratic values in general and free speech concerns in particular. In so doing, they describe how technological paradigms, public policy concerns and legal precedent combined to shape the details of its design. For example, the decision to leave the interactive discussion elements of the network unmoderated owed as much to a concern with avoiding tort liability as it did to a conviction about the democratic value of unmoderated discourse. Overall, Docter and Dutton's chapter provides a shining example of the potential for ICTs to be utilised in pursuit of 'strong democracy', providing that this is the will of those who influence system design.

Conclusion

It is hoped that the contributions to this book go some way towards distinguishing the rhetoric from the reality concerning digital democracy experiments and encourage reflection on the dialectical relationship between technology and society. Whilst the achievements of experiments to date may be somewhat modest, there is every reason to applaud their existence and encourage their development. Anyone concerned with the promotion of 'strong democracy' must be interested in seeking new ways to promote citizen deliberation and build bridges of communication between governments and the governed. ICTs should be seen neither as a panacea for all the ills of democracy nor as the harbingers of a 'Big Brother' state. They should be understood as tools capable of being shaped in the pursuit of radically differing goals, one of which is the achievement of 'strong democracy'.

Notes

1 All the contributors to this collection were free to adopt their own terminology.
2 One such project with which the authors have been closely involved is 'Trimdon Digital Village'. Trimdon is a rural community of 3,050 inhabitants situated in the south of County Durham in the north of England. The digital village project, comprising a local network of three sites with online facilities backed by locally delivered training and support, has the following objectives:

   • to develop an effective community information service system to enhance the economic competitiveness and social well-being of the community of Trimdon;
   • to raise awareness of community informatics applications and their potential for adding economic and social value to rural communities;
   • to provide relevant IT training and skill development to foster innovation and creativity for individual lifelong learning and community prosperity;
   • to establish access to ICTs for as many village inhabitants as possible; and
   • to develop, through action research, appropriate facilitating skills and methodologies that could be used for the more widespread development of community informatics.

The project was underpinned by the following principles. First, the project would attempt to embed the technology into existing community social structures and would try to avoid the temptation of imposing technological solutions upon the community from outside. Second, and relatedly, the project team would comprise members of the community as well as researchers to enable residents to take 'ownership' of the project's development. Third, the researchers, role would be to facilitate and support community decision making. Fourth, the use of existing facilities and social networks would be adopted to foster a flexible multi-site community network. Lastly, a strong partnership at the 'local' level of a broad range of community groups, public, private and voluntary information providers, educational establishments, policy makers and elected representatives, and telecommunications businesses and consultants should be developed. The three sites have been up and running since the summer of 1997 and the project is subject to ongoing evaluation. It is our intention to publish a detailed appraisal in due course.

2 Perspectives on citizen democratisation and alienation in the virtual public sphere

Anna Malina

Introduction

Notions of political freedom and citizenship are rooted in the idea of the public sphere. Whilst commentators over time have defended the media as a sphere of public debate, our traditional media have been accompanied by notions of top down, paternalistic, one-to-many, non-democratic invisibility. Supported by a blend of liberal, communitarian and entrepreneurial philosophies, the emergence of computerised ICTs, known as telematics, has prompted less hierarchical discourses, characterised by the prospect of more intense democratic participation, visible-ness, public-ness and open-ness. Considerable interest centres on possibilities for electronic democracy. National and local governments are attempting to make certain kinds of electronic information more widely available to the public via ICTs. Open list discussions are organised to develop online political discussion, negating the need for participants to share synchronous time and space and permitting more people access to political debates. Random samples of citizens are chosen to participate in deliberative processes designed to augment representative democracy, for example citizen and policy juries. Inputs to parliament and local councils are derived from consensus conferences. In addition, groups organise experiments where different forms of input and output are developed and assessed, e.g. deliberative polling and tele-voting.

Pointing towards the arrival of an information economy, Castells (1995) argues that modern ICTs transform society. He suggests changes similar in magnitude to those initiated by the Industrial Revolution, but qualitatively different to what has gone before. Phil Agre (1997) is not convinced of such close resemblance to the scale of the nineteenth-century upheavals, but he acknowledges the pervasive nature of computer technology and suggests that societal changes should be closely examined. Entrepreneurs in the corporate sector recognise untapped opportunities in markets for new goods and services, and they rush to enfold the new technologies. We also see ICTs designed for entrepreneurial use in the public sector. Some are used to nurture or rejuvenate local cultures and economies and support strategies for sustainable development. Often the networks designed for local purposes also link to a global matrix. So, whilst ICTs can provide a utopian ideal, offering new possibilities for decentralised participation, democracy and citizenship, they can also support extreme centralisation of power. Ensuing struggles for technological advantage can produce a range of different outcomes, bringing huge benefits to some and profound disadvantage to others. The rhetoric that accompanies development of ICTs often provides narrow descriptions of significance, however, constructing a misleading, emancipatory façade that ignores the possibility of side-effects.

In a single chapter of short length, I cannot hope to cover the detailed points that need to be addressed. It would, however, be naïve to ignore certain societal conditions and shaping influences on the design and development of ICTs in capitalist democracies. My intention, therefore, is to move (albeit briefly) between problems of democracy and citizenship; new strategies for emancipatory intervention to rejuvenate the public sphere, i.e. the current political interest in 'community building' and plans to reanimate citizenship and democratic participation; and the ongoing local/global focus on market forces hegemony. As the chapter progresses, intellectual viewpoints useful for exploring the role of ICTs in reshaping the contemporary 'public sphere' link to a variety of theoretical frameworks. 'Habermas's theory of the public sphere', 'concepts of citizenship' 'typologies of democracy', 'technological imperialism', 'geographic utopias' and 'spatial determinism' are each discussed in relation to the opportunities and risks, possibilities and limitations of electronic democracy.

The public sphere (after Habermas)

Philosophically, the concept of the public sphere underpins the idea of communication arenas where 'citizens' are able to participate in democratic processes. Calhoun (1994: 2) suggests that 'a public sphere adequate to a democratic polity depends upon both quality of discourse and quantity of participation'. As Dahlgren (1991: 2) points out, the nature of action in the public sphere is a normative reference point, and a 'visible indicator of our admittedly imperfect democracies'. In 1962, Habermas published a critique of the public sphere (in German), intended to indicate its emancipatory potential and the reasons for its deterioration in capitalist democracies (see Calhoun 1994). When the publication was received in Germany, Habermas was accused of confusing descriptive and normative aspects of the public sphere (Habermas 1994a). Since the English translation in 1989, Habermas has been further accused of neglecting certain very important elements, already well documented elsewhere (e.g. Garnham 1994; Hardt 1996). Still, Habermas (1989) offers an interesting and critical analytical framework of the 'public sphere', in which aspects of social structure, democracy and the role of the media are interwoven in descriptions of particular historical circumstances, encapsulated in the notion of the 'bourgeois public sphere'. As a Marxist with roots in the Frankfurt school of critical thought, he is greatly concerned with the rise of the culture industry, bureaucratisation and commodification of social life.

In his critique, Habermas describes the way in which early 'public' opinion was socially formed by (only) one public: the eighteenth-century European bourgeoisie, a group of privileged and powerful men, private individuals who constituted themselves as 'the public', and engaged in 'face-to-face' communicative action in critical judgement of public authority. This elite openly discussed political issues in a space set apart from the state and civil society. The formation of 'public opinion' was said to emerge as a direct outcome of 'rational–critical debate'. This is where Habermas conceptualises an 'ideal' of the 'public sphere' (not yet realised) that supports widespread, undistorted, face-to-face communication.

There is a clear distinction between social and economic arenas. To constitute 'social integration', the realm of interaction is specifically a 'social' sphere, termed 'lifeworld', that operates outside the machinations of money and power. 'System integration, on the other hand, wholly depends on and generates money and power. Tracing a historical path, Habermas illustrates a 'precarious balance' between 'lifeworld' and 'system' organisations up until the mid-twentieth century (see McGuigan 1996), when the public sphere was transformed historically by a combination of social changes, e.g. industrialisation, the growth of literacy and the development of a 'protective' welfare state (see Dahlgren 1991). By the early twentieth century, an interventionist bureaucratic state had arrived and escalation of the capitalist media increasingly supported social engineering, e.g. public relations and advertising (see Mayhew 1997). Differences between public and private in political and economic domains were blurred, shifting the focus from rational discussion of politics and culture to mass consumerism. Instrumental 'colonisation' of the lifeworld by capitalist systems resulted in the 'aggrandisement' of capitalism. As a result, human values and the quest for meaning in the lifeworld were subjugated by systemic imperatives that were not compelled to uphold moral questions of human value and meaning (McGuigan 1996). When rational–critical debate was blocked, the public sphere became dysfunctional, and at this point, Habermas claims, it gradually fell into decline.

Habermas (1989) points to the ability of modern propaganda methods to construct illusion, thus producing many different side-effects. Professional expertise able to create ideational content to order can be purchased on the open market by already powerful groups. Thus biased and manipulated representations pervade all areas of our lives and communicative practices, thwarting meaningful communication. The clear warning from Habermas is that the constant pursuit of profit by the capitalist media, the increasing importance of mass consumerism, and the rise of certain types of institutional power – aided by professional persuasion – are destroying meaningful public communication.

In fact, Habermas now concedes, markets and bureaucracies are necessary in complex capitalist societies. In addition, critical theory recognises that private interests are often developed in the 'public sphere'. Habermas is concerned with the ideal as well as the reality, however, and whilst his discourses operate at a high level of abstraction, the descriptions he offers stress normative aspects of communication media and the problem of organising open democratic expression in the public sphere.

Nowadays, the potential of widespread communicative action and principles relating to individualism, self-fulfilment and the ability to create our own identities are cited as important elements in the development and design of new roles for modern ICTs. Many point to the fresh possibilities for autonomous expression offered by easier access to an electronically mediated public sphere. Joshua Meyrowitz (1985) argues that new electronic media have 'clouded the difference between stranger and friend', suggesting that new forms of human emotion are beginning to evolve from interactions in multiple discussion groups. This observation is markedly different to the involvement of only one 'elite' public in the Habermasian formulation of the public sphere, and highlights the interaction within distinct groups and between people belonging to different publics and oppositional groupings.

Notions of collective participation and the language of 'community' are also central to the development of new roles for ICTs. Virtual communitarian Howard Rheingold (1993) maintains an optimistic philosophy as he outlines positive outcomes of sustained cultural activity and political action in 'shared communities'. Rheingold describes a radical revitalisation of the public sphere, explaining that electronic networks have allowed people to interact locally or transcend borders to exchange information and share common interests in interactive forums – multiple 'public spheres' that he calls 'virtual communities'. When discussion groups are developed, each forum is a public sphere in its own right, offering the opportunity for direct participation. Rheingold maintains that there is immense potential for democratic outcomes. Arguing that democracy and technology affect one another, he rejuvenates the idea of a 'social commons', and highlights new possibilities for the social order, even suggesting that public electronic networks (PENs) represent a new form of 'digital democracy' as a result of their emphasis on citizen-to-citizen communication.

Technologies do not just happen, however; according to Sclove, they are 'contingent social products' (Sclove 1995: 7). That is, one design is chosen over another and development is influenced by prevailing norms, beliefs and social structures. Whilst other designs are always possible, citizens are increasingly urged to use ICTs routinely billed as emancipatory. Those ICTs used ostensibly for emancipatory purposes can also support structures that represent anti-democratic formations. Development is dependent on which set of beliefs is most dominant. Where democratic outcomes are detected, prevailing forces that influenced the design of new roles for ICTs are also likely to be democratic. Nevertheless, human contexts remain mutable, and in settings where other forces are more dominant, different inputs and outcomes are likely to ensue.

Globalisation indicates the ease with which national borders are breached by social, cultural, political and economic processes. Currently, it is widely claimed that electronic commerce is growing. With more people connected to speedy forms of information and communication, there are increasing opportunities for developing, selling and buying services anywhere in the world. Large-scale commercial service providers sell access to a virtual world of fast, easy, electronic information and communication. On entry to commercial zones, customers are assembled at the electronic portals. Subsequent movement between links is mediated by the mercantile nature of virtual architecture. Already captive audiences inside a commercially mediated maze are easily bombarded with advertising appeals. Problems here are not so much related to issues of access or social inclusion/exclusion; misgivings lie more with the difficulty of moving outside heavily commercialised sectors. Concerns also arise from the mistaken assumption that interactivity in all electronic arenas, however trivial or overtly commercial, is somehow commensurate with empowerment and democratic participation in the 'electronic public sphere'.

The worth of the public sphere is dependent on the accessibility and adequacy of information and communication. Schiller (1996: xi) is concerned about the nature of media information, controlled by a market forces hegemony that invariably concentrates on presenting trivia and 'sensationalist material' and largely ignores important social and political issues. Moreover, information can be packaged as 'social good' openly and freely available, or as 'privately produced commodity for sale' (Schiller 1996: 35). Entrepreneurial institutions and companies detect lucrative new markets. They organise or buy information, store it electronically and later sell on to those who can afford to pay. Even if the principle of universal access to ICTs is established, need to pay means that expensive and highly sought-after information is restricted to those who can afford to pay the charges. Already, only rich institutions, cities, businesses and individuals are able to buy the most highly priced information, and so accrue immense advantages for themselves in the market-place. Conversely, an inability to pay large amounts of money prevents access to the best information, relegating the poorest consumers to an exclusion zone, a 'cyber-ghetto', where only inferior information is cheap enough for budget restrictions.

Nevertheless, a mask of democracy is detectable in the emancipatory discourses surrounding new ICTs, often billed as able to provide better information and the opportunity for wider publics in civil society to be involved in political discussions. In reality, however, emancipatory outcomes are not certain in liberal protective democracies, where Held (1987: 98) points out that state politics are separate from civil society – considered the sphere of the 'economy, culture and family life'. In state politics, there is a general focus on private ownership of the means of production and development of a competitive market economy (Held 1987: 99). It seems likely that the unequal gaps that already exist between rich and poor in civil society will widen dramatically if ICTs are designed primarily in support of information held as privately owned property for sale in a highly commercialised and competitive 'electronic' public sphere.

To ignore the ramifications of ICTs is negligent, Sclove argues, for in doing so we risk indifference to the way in which they can be organised to support different power relations in the public sphere. Whilst recognising that there are very few ways in which citizens can influence the process of choosing or designing technologies, we should not 'adapt compliantly to whatever technologies happen along', but commit ourselves to supporting technologies that are 'compatible' with citizenship and democracy (Sclove 1995: 8–9).

'Concepts of citizenship' and 'typologies of democracy'

Citizens acquire rights and are protected by state power in return for performing certain duties for the state. The nature of these rights and duties emerges from a contract between the nation-state and its members (Webster 1996: 68), and the urge to create more equality is considered the constant goal of democratic societies that remain open to change (Held 1993). Whilst T.H. Marshall confers 'equal rights and duties, liberties, constraints, powers and responsibilities on citizens' (Marshall 1973: 84), many 'publics' in societies that have claimed democratic cultures have missed out on entitlements. Even classical Athenian democracy – often upheld as an ideal – restricted the entitlement of citizenship to relatively small numbers of people who were selected from the whole public and allocated certain rights, whilst the rest were largely excluded. Whilst the term 'public' is often taken to mean the whole community and citizenship, many people, including women, ethnic groups and the lower classes, have often been denied rights of citizenship and communication. According to Habermas, it is an 'imprecise linguistic term' when used in phrases such as 'public interest' or 'public sphere'. In principle the 'public sphere' is available on a universal scale, but in reality the language of universalism does not always translate into open access to the means of communication for everyone (Habermas 1994b).

'Socialists in the Marxist tradition' believe 'that the language of universalism masks unequal power stemming from unequal relations in civil society' (Meehan 1994: 78). Meehan further suggests that, for Marxists, citizenship is attached to ownership of property, and unequal ownership indicates unequal citizenship. Inequality promotes a view of the citizen as subject. On the other hand, proponents of the welfare state suggest that, with proper intervention, unequal citizenship need not result. Even so, liberal democracy in the UK –

influenced by Schumpeter's low estimation of the average citizen – evolved particular notions of citizenship that have drawn away from the ideal goals described by T.H. Marshall. Increased bureaucratisation and class relations in civil society created an unequal distribution of political power; and the notion of citizenship became more closely entwined with property ownership and the concept of moral fitness.

The practice of politics does not escape public notice, and as rightwing neo-liberalism continued to develop along asymmetrical lines, the public began to indicate distrust of traditional politics. By the early 1990s, just as a 'wave of democracy' swept across several countries beyond the West (Markoff 1996), it was argued that public trust in liberal democracy and other traditional structures was declining in the UK (Hall and Jacques 1990). Politicians appeared to be losing power, not least because of their perceived inability to understand major public problems escalated by sweeping societal changes (see McGrew 1997). Some (e.g. Wright 1994) argued that democracy not only needed to be taken more seriously, it needed to be radically overhauled and modernised.

Developments here influenced and were no doubt influenced by the immense transformations that contemporary societies have undergone in recent decades (see Hall *et al.* 1993). The high cost of dealing with the effects of social problems and increased fear of anomie, which Durkheim explains as normlessness resulting from rapid social change, promotes a new focus on social inclusion, now thought necessary to reconstruct societies and make them more cohesive. By the late 1990s, the idea of 'community' was central to what modernising protagonists of New Labour's 'third way' termed 'social investment'. Here, sociologist Anthony Giddens points to a policy move away from 'market fundamentalism' towards a 'mixed economy', where the aim is to strike a better balance between economic and non-economic areas of social life (Giddens 1998: 18–21). Combining elements from liberal and Marxist traditions, the UK's Labour government now attempts to increase democratic autonomy, favouring a more participatory democracy. Democratic autonomy suggests that people should be free and equal to determine the conditions of their own life, and Held's 'principle(s) of justification' for 'participatory democracy', suggests that:

> [A]n equal right to liberty and self-development can only be achieved in a 'participatory society', a society which fosters a sense of political efficacy, nurtures a concern for collective prob-

lems and contributes to the formation of a knowledgeable citizenry capable of taking a sustained interest in the governing process.

(Held 1987: 271)

Held refers to the work of Pateman, who draws from Rousseau and J.S. Mill to argue that participatory democracy sustains human development (Held 1987). Whilst there is an awareness that the ordinary person is unlikely to maintain interest in all political discussions, it is expected that people will be concerned about processes that directly affect their own lives. Citizens, therefore, should be enabled to exert some power and control over events at the local level. However, the liberal focus on political representation, a competitive multiparty system and elections are considered unavoidable, and they are likely, therefore, to remain central to participatory democracy (Held 1987).

New strategies aim to produce a socially responsible, educated citizenry and to create a more egalitarian capitalism. Local governments are pressurised to accept responsibility for quality of life in their locality and at the same time they are to be made more accessible and transparent. Experimentation with political forms and development of new liberatory roles for modern ICTs is endorsed. When they are designed specifically for the purpose, ICTs are able to provide better information and communication, thus supporting participatory democracy's goal to improve the 'poor resource base of social groups' and sustain 'direct participation of citizens in the regulation of the key institutions of society, including the workplace and local community' (Held 1987: 271).

Whilst ICTs can be designed to help realise formally recognised citizen liberties, freedom requires a common and 'effective moral basis', Sclove argues, to support the design of more democratic technologies and a system of active electronic participation. To embrace democratic roles, technologies need to accommodate the tenets of 'strong democracy'. Following Kantian moral philosophy, people must respect one another's needs, and be prepared to act on behalf of the common good. As Giddens (1994a) points out, everyone is involved to some extent in affecting society, and we all constantly endorse or alter societal conditions. Sclove (1995: 35) takes the basic concept of 'structuration' (Giddens 1979) – that we are all shaped by structure and action in routine activities – and proposes that we 'should be guided by an overarching respect for moral freedom' when designing ICTs for democratic purposes. He uses the term 'democratic structuration' to situate this explanatory concept in a 'normative context'.

To describe the nature of democratic thought critically, Held (1987) constructs four classic models of democracy: classical democracy, protective democracy, development democracy and direct democracy, and five contemporary models: contemporary-elitist democracy, pluralism, legal democracy, participatory democracy and democratic autonomy. Van Dijk (1996) elaborates the first four of Held's (1987) contemporary models, replacing democratic autonomy with plebiscitary democracy. Connecting these models to the practice of democracy via ICTs, van Dijk finds that 'the goals and means of designing and using ICT in the political system can be very different' (1996: 54). He suggests that some groups seek to 'preserve the current system of democracy' because they view utopian goals as dangerous (van Dijk 1996: 43), and he warns that ICTs might be designed to 'reinforce institutional politics' and 'revive the steering ambitions within states' (van Dijk 1996: 55). Ideal concepts of democracy and citizenship do not indicate actually existing routines – they are goals not yet realised – and van Dijk suggests that explicit compromises can be made in the construction of democracy, drawing from different models to further the positive use of ICTs in democratic action.

Tony Held suggests that it has now become important to examine the potential for more direct participatory democracy, because technically people can now vote electronically, choosing those they want to elect to office from a range of competing political parties and voting in direct relation to legislative procedures. Fast action, interactive, push-button facilities can now link to electronic campaigns, databases and registers, and tele-referenda, tele-polling and electronic elections are used in many different experimental political processes. Budge (1996: 1) proposes that the 'challenge of direct democracy is to the limited participation of citizens in their own government'. Hacker and Todino (1996) discuss alternative types of political participation using ICTs, clearly differentiating between the concepts of 'electronic democracy' and 'electronic democratisation'. 'Electronic democracy' is considered to be the ability to provide practical means, i.e. the provision of instruments such as 'electronic townhalls', which bypass more traditional routes. Electronic features provide a higher degree of citizen involvement in the political process through push-button voting and tele-referenda. 'Electronic democracy', therefore, has some similarity with 'plebiscitary democracy', which endorses the sum of individual opinion.

Populist politician Ross Perot describes a dream vision of an 'electronic agora', a 'technological utopia' where a new era of direct democracy results from electronically recording responses. There is little to indicate, however, that people will want to be involved in this way, or that they will sustain participation over time. Arterton (1987) is not confident that such responses will develop. Moreover, what this kind of political rhetoric fails to explain is that choices do not always take account of minority needs, and responses can easily be limited in the way in which pre-set criteria are assembled. In addition, voters may be overwhelmed with information, constrained by time and unable to understand the complex issues at stake, particularly when subjected to the political manoeuvring of media specialists.

Abramson *et al.* (1988) believe that the emphasis on plebiscites can quicken democracy but that it can simultaneously inhibit the practice of slower, more deliberative, forms of democracy, where different views can be presented and discussed rationally before well-reasoned judgements are made. Thompson (1995: 258) too suggests that deliberative democracy is not 'best served' by the arrival of the 'electronic town hall' or other forms of tele-democracy. In Thompson's view, the reasoned judgement of all ordinary people should be valued and incorporated into decision-making processes at different levels of social and political life.

Electronic democratisation, as Hacker and Todino (1996: 72) explain, is the means of enhancing processes of democracy already assumed to be in place, in ways that 'increase the political power of those whose role in key political processes is usually minimised'. The organisation of citizen juries linked to ICTs can be useful here. In order to conceptualise electronic democratisation in the first place, however, certain suppositions about democracy must be made explicit, e.g.

> [f]irst democracy involves responsiveness of governments and leaders to the concerns and preferences of its citizens; second, that leaders and citizens are political equals; and third that citizen preferences are weighted with no discrimination by content or source of preference.
>
> (Hacker and Todino 1996: 71)

'Technological imperialism', 'geographic utopias' and spatial determinism'

Political benefits of ICT promoted for the common good are often stressed by capitalist governments. At the same time, information and communication are viewed as vital commodities. As Feldman points out, 'digital information' is 'manipulable', 'networkable', 'dense', 'compressible' and 'impartial' (Feldman 1997: 3), and these key features underpin the importance of contemporary ICTs and electronic communication. There are massive advantages for those able to control the flow of electronic information. Together with more flexible means of communication, control of information is a necessary component of cultural domination, and there is immense economic interest in production, dissemination and consumption of communication. In 1972, UNESCO drew the world's attention to the way in which media sourced in rich countries were able to dominate cultures and world opinion, and we now see evidence of 'technological imperialism', where producers of digital products are embroiled in conflict, busily developing lucrative new global markets to sell a varied and constantly changing range of IT-related products. When need is established, ICTs are developed as a highly profitable source of power and wealth. Ever more sophisticated technological features permit many-to-many communication, and offer the potential for unlimited human interaction. Whilst citizenship may be improved and state power enhanced by the development of ICTs, Schiller (1996) suggests that the main beneficiaries are large global corporations. Huge corporate activities stretch divisions *'between'* and *'within'* countries, and the gap widens even further between the well-off and disadvantaged locally and globally (Schiller 1996: 104).

According to Castells (1995), ICTs have had such a direct instrumental impact on society and the economy that they have produced patterns of change in information processing that give rise to a new information economy. Although the notion of a fully fledged information economy is in dispute, there is little doubt that there is a growing political and economic focus on developing a local/global communications infrastructure. Already, many hurriedly seek reorganisation of their information and communication structures. Castells (1995) argues that the organisational and institutional use of information technology (IT) alters bureaucracies and signifies an important, though complex, technological change to the 'mode of production' in cities and regions. He highlights Saskia Sassen's notion

that global cities and local regions are now taking on more responsible economic roles, drawing away from the importance of the
nation-state. Information City initiatives encourage growth and stim-
ulation of electronic spaces for public and private interaction.
ICTs considered relevant to cultural and economic developments in
poor, marginalised areas prompt the rise of urban regeneration
community development initiatives that aim to rejuvenate geographic
locales.

These approaches to distinct urban conditions show recognition
of the sharp differences between rich and poor, who live in very
different areas of the same city. What Castells (1995) describes as
the 'dual city', houses the urban poor in poverty stricken 'ghetto'
areas and the extremely rich in highly affluent districts. Whilst divisions in wealth have long been discernible in cities, Castells argues,
an information economy dramatically escalates the growing dispar-
ities between different income groups and geographic areas. Cultural
and economic differences widen as a result of different routine experiences and wide variations in income. The information city's rich
IT workers interact locally and globally, often routinely orbiting the
earth via sophisticated ICTs during the course of a day's work. They
are often 'cosmopolitan' in outlook and have the financial ability
to travel anywhere in the world. The urban poor, on the other hand,
tend to think and act locally, often lacking motivation and constricted
by an economic inability to travel far from home (Castells, 1995;
Webster 1996).

The concepts of 'time–space distanciation' (Giddens 1994b) and
'time space compression' (Harvey 1989) draw attention to the elas-
ticity of time and space and the ability of speedy forms of
communication to dissembed one set of cultural meanings and re-
embed those significations suited to the most powerful hegemonic
influences. As new ICTs become more efficient and widely used,
'distanciated relations' are extended, and people and events from far
outside an area can easily influence what is happening in a locality
(see Giddens 1994b; Allen and Hamnett 1995). Local entrepreneurs
are needed inside the area to interpret and represent interests from
outside the locality, and a mediated system of local interaction at
different levels can help to establish trust in new conditions (Lash
and Urry 1994: 284).

Castells suggests that organisational management in urban areas
is 'decentralised', whilst 'high level decision making' is increasingly
'centralised'; but the importance is the relationship between them by
means of 'communication flows' (Castells 1995: 169). Centralised

systems are increasingly dependent on customised delivery of services and retrieval of information, whilst decentralised systems await instructions from the top. Each requires connection to a 'corresponding level of the communication network', thus elevating the importance of spatial logic in the economy (Castells 1995: 169). Decentralisation of responsibility does not, however, mean complete freedom at the local level; instead, local structures provide a flexible supportive mechanism for centralised power (Robins and Webster 1988).

Southern (1997: 11) claims that the broadening of the term 'electronic democracy' has 'dovetailed' into the 'operations of the public sector', which has 'taken on board the potential of information technology'. Assumptions woven into the discourses around ICTs invoke what might be termed 'spatial determinism', underpinning a notion that society and culture are ruled by the ability of ICTs to solve problems by conquering space. Often the rhetoric used venerates network technology, highlighting a liberatory capacity to enlarge benefits greatly for people in geographic areas.

Growth in the sale of ICTs can be attached to successful promotion of their worth in the marketplace. Utopian assumptions about ICTs, along with policy and marketing initiatives that drive their development, combine with grassroots efforts mobilised to muster assets and defend local space and a tribal need to maintain identity. Impelled by these very different forces, cities increasingly spawn expensive 'quick fix' technological initiatives for community development, without full knowledge of the limits or side-effects of the technology used. Some cities feel that they will 'miss out' if they do not quickly acquire new ICTs and adapt to their use. Thus, ICTs are implemented to gain crucial social and economic advantages for well-off areas, and technological answers to social, cultural and economic problems in poorer, marginalised areas. Even if the technology fails to be utilised to its full potential to improve outcomes, the appearance alone of 'high-tech' can be advantageous. An advanced ICT system can greatly enhance place image and attract positive attention to areas.

The development of ICTs is to be market driven and led by the private sector, and many city councils are committed to building public–private alliances to develop ICTs and promote urban entrepreneurialism (see Malina and Jankowski 1998). The tendency over time for public and private interests to overlap is intensifying further, and partnerships develop new caring moral values and a co-operative approach to communication strategies geared for the integration of local, regional and national economies in a global system. Partnerships also address existing civic decay and combat high levels of crime and other social and economic problems experienced in less affluent areas. Whilst community building is community based and community developed, directed at collective culture and general well-being for all, individual citizens are not always consulted or directly involved during the design of locally based ICTs for that purpose. Instead, social, civic and commercial sectors invest in the community partnership and harness social and economic capital on behalf of local people to address problems and improve community life.

Citizens are, however, involved directly as a source of labour. The process of skilling a service workforce is already in development. People are informed that they must take on the responsibility for developing new skills. A notion of the 'learning society' is being underlined, and catch-phrases like 'learning from cradle to grave' attempt to inspire an active spirit of learning. Economically, it makes good sense in a rapidly changing world of electronic communication to sustain a dynamic workforce who practise lifelong learning; moreover, new types of skills are often required for a higher level of labour. Opposite to the logic of Fordism, less affluent workers must develop the intellectual potential to cope with the nature of information work, which often demands a level of problem-solving ability. Of course, any new knowledge gained can be used in civic as well as work contexts.

Some of those who must return to learning find larger educational institutions alienating. This is where locally designed electronic networks can be helpful in co-ordinating the delivery of skilling programmes implemented at the grassroots level by more familiar local groups utilising local access sites such as pubs, clubs, schools and community centres for the purpose. Cultural identity must also be altered so that citizens become aware of their own economic importance in the development of local areas and communities currently being shaped as appropriate production sites for local and global service industries. It is hoped that benefits will 'trickle down' later to the individual citizen.

A focus on geographic utopias and a new local workforce supports the structural adjustments that will weave ICTs more firmly into civil society and at the same time establish shared cultural and economic routines. ICTs developed at the local level can be designed to meet the needs and demands of patrons situated inside and outside the locale. Whilst the initial intention is for local activities to become more robust and so enhance localised institutional routines, local commerce and the life-chances of local citizens, the infrastructure (still in design) can also support centralised forces, e.g. national, international, transnational and global hegemonies.

Conclusion: democratisation and alienation

Whilst the use of ICTs to improve democracy is often overstated, technology used innovatively in pursuit of the ideal is not inconsequential, and where the seeds of strong democracy exist, ICTs can extend and broaden positive aspects of democratic practice. The possibilities for electronic democratisation are, however, dependent on whether the appropriate information is packaged as an easily accessible 'social good' or sold as a costly 'consumer product'. Outcomes are also relative to the typology of democracy practised and the perceptions of citizenship held. Where normative aspects and genuine democratic practice are absent, and where citizens are held in low regard or excluded by their representatives and other experts in the public sphere, outcomes for democratic autonomy, more participatory democracy and social cohesion will be gloomy. As Mayhew (1997: 81) points out, social integration 'must be founded on the legitimate social relations that people undertake to form cultures, build character, and collectively resolve social problems'. A bias towards representative and expert involvement can blur opportunities for ordinary members of the public to become involved in democratic practices. Shapiro (1994) acknowledges the value of expertise, but suggests – as Hacker and Todino (1996: 79) put it – that experts should not be allowed 'to monopolise key decision-making processes'; rather, a theory of democracy indicates the need to: 'empower the disempowered, extend the boundaries of political debate, make enfranchisement into the system of political discourse easier, make political discourse more rational and informative, and bring citizens closer to interaction with centres of power' (Hacker and Todino 1996: 79).

Important cultural and economic freedoms can be extended in the local electronic public sphere as a result of ICTs designed by a combination of local people and experts specifically for that purpose. This chapter ends, however, with the notion that local potential capitalised – albeit compassionately – into market values by social, civic and economic entrepreneurs constituted in partnership is likely to support institutional and economic hegemonies, and to skew the features of electronic democracy towards an increasingly centralised and highly competitive global market agenda.

3 Democracy and cyberspace

Richard K. Moore

Digital cyberspace: a quick tour of the future

Let's stand back for a moment from today's internet and from the temporary lag in deployment of state-of-the-art digital technology. From a longer perspective, certain aspects of the future cyberspace are plain to see.

As regards transport infrastructure – the pipes – cyberspace is simply the natural and inevitable integration/rationalisation of the disparate, patched-together, special-purpose networks that make up the nervous system of modern societies. Besides the public distribution systems such as terrestrial and satellite broadcast, cable and telephone (cellular and otherwise), this integration will also extend to dedicated private systems, such as those that handle point-of-sale transactions, tickets and reservations, inter-bank transfers, CCTV surveillance, stock transfers, etc.

The cost savings, performance gains and application flexibility brought by such total integration are simply too compelling for this integration scenario to be seriously doubted. Just as surely as the telegraph replaced the carrier pigeon, and the telephone replaced the telegraph, this integration is one bit of progress that is bound to happen, one way or another, sooner or later.

Significant technical work is still required on the infrastructure, to provide efficiently and reliably such mandatory features as security, guaranteed bandwidth, accountability, authentication, and the prevention of 'mail-bombs' and other internet anomalies. These features do not, however, require rocket science – they are more a matter of selecting from proven technologies and agreeing on standards, interconnect arrangements and implementation schedules.

The global digital high-bandwidth network – the hardware of cyberspace – will in fact be the ultimate distribution mechanism for the mass-media industry: it will subsume broadcast (air and cable) television, video-tape rentals, and perhaps even audio CDs. These familiar niceties will go the way of vinyl records and punched cards.

Cyberspace will be the universal connection of the individual to the world at large: 'transactions on the net' will be the way to access funds and accounts, make purchases and reservations, pay taxes, view media products (films, news, sports, entertainment, etc.), initiate real-time calls, send and receive messages from individuals and groups, query traffic-congestion patterns, etc. *ad infinitum*. Each transaction will have an associated price, posted to your account, with some portion going to the ultimate vendor (e.g. content provider) and some going to the various intermediaries – just as with credit card purchases today.

Today's internet: democratised communications

Today's internet is most remarkable for its cultural aspects. Technically, the internet is one small episode in the ever-evolving parade of technology, soon to be outmoded. Culturally and economically, however, the internet seems to be a phenomenon nearly unprecedented in human history.

The internet is a non-monetised communications realm, an open global commons, a communications marketplace with a very special economics in both content and transport. Each physical node (and its connecting hook-ups) is, in essence, donated to the network infrastructure by its operator (government agency, private company, university, ISP) for his or her own and the common benefit – a classic case of anarchistic mutual benefit. Similarly, the content of the internet is a voluntary commons: anyone can be a publisher or can self-publish their own work. Publications of all levels of quality and subject matter are available, generally for free. The only costs to a user are typically fixed and moderate. Everyone in the globe is a local call away, so to speak, and communication with groups is as cheap and convenient as communication with individuals.

Anyone can join the global internet co-op for a modest fee. The internet brings the massification of discourse; it prototypes the democratisation of media. Individuals voluntarily serve as 'intelligent agents', forwarding on items of interest to various groups. Web sites bristle with links to related sites, and an almost infinite world of information becomes effectively accessible even by novices.

Netizens experience this global commons as a democratic renaissance, a flowering of public discourse, a finding-of-voice by millions who would otherwise have had no available means of public expression. Like-minded people can virtually gather together, across national boundaries and without concern for time-zones. Information, perhaps published in an obscure leaflet in an unknown corner of the world, is suddenly brought to the attention of thousands worldwide – based on its intrinsic interest-value.

The net is especially effective in the co-ordination of real-world organisations – enhancing group communication, reducing travel and meetings, and enabling more rapid decision making. The real-world political impact of internet culture up to now is difficult to gauge. Interesting and powerful ideas are discussed online – infinitely broader than what occurs in mass-media 'public discourse' – but to a large extent such ideas seem buried in the net itself, and when the computer is turned off one wonders if it wasn't all just a dream, confined to the ether. So far, there seems to be minimal spillover into the real world.

Ironically, at least from my perspective, it seems to be right-wing organisations that are making most effective political use of the net at present – organising write-in campaigns, mobilising opinion around focused issues, etc. Those of us with more liberal democratic values seem more divided and less driven to achieving actual concrete results. One wonders, however, what might happen if a period of popular activism were to occur, such as we saw in the 1960s, the 1930s, 1900s, 1848, 1798, 1776, etc. If a similar episode of unrest were to recur, the internet might turn out to be a sleeping political giant – co-ordinating protests, facilitating strategy discussions, mobilising massive voter turnouts, distributing reports suppressed in the mass media, etc. The 'people's' mass media could have an awesome effect on the body politic, if some motivating urgency were to crystallise activism.

Such a scenario is not just idle imagining. Eruptions of activism do in fact occur (there have been a few in Germany, France and Australia recently, for example). The net is not yet widespread enough to have been significant in such events (as far as I know), but we may be very close to critical mass in some Western countries, and the power of the internet for real-world group organisation has been tested and proven.

This activist–empowerment potential of the internet is something that many elements of society would naturally find very threatening. Some countries, such as Iran, China and Malaysia – where 'motivating urgency' exists in the populous – take the threat of 'excess democracy' quite seriously, and have instituted various kinds of

restrictive internet policies. I would presume – and this point will
be developed a bit later – that awareness (in ruling circles) of the
'subversive' threat from the internet lends considerable political
support to the various net-censorship initiatives that are underway
in Western nations, and that such awareness may largely explain
the mass-media image of the internet as a land of hackers, terrorists and paedophiles.

Partly because of this potential activist 'threat', and partly because
of economic considerations, there is considerable reason to suspect
that the internet culture will not long continue quite as we know
it. Apart from censorship itself, chilling copyright and libel laws,
and other measures, are in the works that can in various direct and
indirect ways close the damper on the open internet. The average
Joe Citizen, spoon-fed by the mass media, all too often holds the
opinion that the internet is a haven of perverts and terrorists, and
thus internet restrictions are not met with the same public outcry
that would accompany, for example, newspaper censorship.

The internet offers a prototype demonstration of how cyberspace
could be applied to enhance the democratic process – to make it
more open and participatory. Netizens are not the only ones with
their eyes on the cyberspace prize, however, and we next examine
another potential cyberspace client – the mass-media industry.

The mass media: monopolised communications

Like the internet, today's mass-media industry is also a global
communications network, and also offers access to seemingly infinite information. Beyond these similarities, however, the two could
not be more different: whilst internet exchange is non-economic,
mass media is increasingly fully commercialised; whilst anyone can
publish on the net, publication access to mass media is controlled
by those who own it; whilst the full spectrum of public thinking
can be found on the net, discussion in the mass media is narrow
and systematically projects the world-view of its owners.

In the mass media, rather than voluntary contributors, we have
'content owners' and 'content producers'. Instead of free mailing-
lists, web links, and voluntary forwarding agents, we have 'content
distributors' – including broadcast networks, cable operators, satellite operators, cinema chains, and video rental chains; and instead
of an audience of participants or netizens, we have 'consumers'.

In both networks, the information content reflects the interests of
the owners. With the internet, this means that the content is as

broad as society itself; but with the mass media, the narrow scope of content reflects the fact that ownership of mass media, on a global scale, is increasingly coming to be concentrated in a clique of large corporate conglomerates. The mass media does not serve discourse, education or democracy particularly well; it is designed instead to distribute corporate-approved products to 'consumers', and to manage public opinion.

The US telecom and media industries have long been privatised, and hence the corporatised version of mass media is most thoroughly evolved in the US. It is the US model that, for the most part, seems destined to become the global norm – partly because the US provides a microcosmic precedent of what are becoming global conditions (a corporate-dominated economy), and partly because the US effectively promulgates its pro-corporate policies in international forums.

As state-run broadcasting systems are increasingly privatised under globalisation, it is the deep-pockets corporate media operators who are likely to acquire them, thus propagating the US media model globally, although US operators will by no means be the only buyers in the market.

The US model is a monopoly model. a 'clique of majors' dominates the industry, just as the Seven-Sisters clique dominates the world oil market. *The Nation*, 3rd June 1996, published a remarkable road-map of the US news and entertainment industry, graphically highlighting the collective hegemony of GE, Time-Warner, Disney-Cap-Cities, and Westinghouse. These majors are vertically integrated, i.e. they own not only production facilities and content, but also distribution systems, radio and television broadcast stations, satellites, cable systems and cinema chains.

We might think of Time-Warner and Disney as being primarily media companies, but for GE and Westinghouse, media is clearly a side-line business. They are into everything from nuclear power-stations and jet fighters, to insurance and medical equipment. Their broadcast policies reflect not only the profit motive of their media companies but equally the overall interests of the owning conglomerate. NBC is not likely, for example, to run an exposé of GE nuclear-reactor safety problems or of corruption involving GE's government contracts.

When you consider the ownership of the mass media, and the additional influence of corporate advertisers, it is no surprise that the content of mass media – not just news but entertainment as well – overwhelmingly projects a world-view that is friendly to corporate interests generally.

As globalisation proceeds, these four conglomerates – along with Rupent Murdoch and others – will compete to buy up distribution and production facilities on a worldwide basis. The clear trend, following a shake-out period, is towards a global mass-media industry dominated by a clique of TNC (transnational corporation) 'majors'. The globalisation of the media industry translates ultimately into corporate domination of global information flows, and the centralised management of global public opinion.

Whereas the internet precedent suggests the potential of cyberspace to connect citizens with one another on a participatory basis, a corporate-dominated mass-media industry sees cyberspace primarily as a product distribution system and a means of opinion-control. In order to assess how cyberspace will in fact be applied, we need to examine the political context in which cyberspace will evolve; we need to take a closer look at this thing called 'democracy'.

The see-saw of democracy and the advent of globalisation

Democracy has always been a see-saw struggle for control between citizens at large and elite economic interests. This struggle has been perhaps more apparent in a country like Britain, where a consciously acknowledged class system long operated. In the US, with its more egalitarian rhetoric, there has often been a tendency to deny the existence of such struggles and to embrace the mythology that popular sovereignty has been largely achieved in the 'land of the free'.

In fact, the tension between popular and elite interests was anticipated by America's Founding Fathers, was articulated explicitly by James Madison (primary architect of the US Constitution) and was institutionalised in that document by the balance between the Senate and the House of Representatives, and by numerous other means.

Under democracy, power is officially vested in the voters, and hence the balance of power between the elite and the people would seem to be overwhelmingly in favour of the people. For their part, the economic elite have considerable influence due to the investments and credit they control and the funds they have available to influence the political process in various and significant ways. Hence the balance of power is not that easy to call, and there has in fact been a see-saw of power shifts over the past two centuries. During the late nineteenth-century 'robber baron' era, for example, with its *laissez-faire* philosophy, there was a clear predominance of elite power, with monopolised markets and widespread worker exploitation. In the reform movements of the early twentieth century, on the other hand, with its trust-busting and regulatory regimes, the elite found themselves on the defensive.

In today's world of neoliberal globalisation, the economic elite are again clearly in the ascendancy. The vehicle of elite power and ownership today is the modern TNC, and globalisation – with its privatisation, deregulation, lower corporate taxes, and free-trade policies – adds up to a radical shift of power and assets from the nation-state (where the democratic see-saw operates) to TNCs, over which citizens have no significant influence (the campaigns of Ralph Nader, Greenpeace, *et al.* having been systematically constrained and marginalised).

Economic policy making, which has traditionally fallen under the jurisdiction of sovereign nation-states, is being transferred wholesale by various treaties to the WTO (World Trade Organisation), the IMF and other faceless commissions – all of which are dominated overwhelmingly by the TNC community, particularly by that clique of TNCs known as the 'international financial community'.

This transfer of economic sovereignty is most advanced in the Third World, where the IMF increasingly dictates economic, fiscal and social policies at a micro level. In India, for example, public officials often turn directly to IMF staff for policy guidance, leaving the Indian government out of the loop entirely.

The trends, and the binding treaty commitments, indicate that the First World as well is destined to come under increasing domination by this TNC run, globalist commission regime. Already we are beginning to see examples of such inroads, as US policy towards Cuba is being challenged under NAFTA, and EU beef import policy is being challenged under the WTO, along with market protections for Caribbean banana producers. These examples are only the tip of the formidable globalist iceberg lying in the path of the once sovereign Ship of State.

Globalisation amounts to a *coup d'état* by the global economic elite. Temporary political ascendancy in the West is being systematically leveraged into permanent, global, political ascendancy, institutionalised in the network of elite-dominated commissions and agencies. The see-saw game has been abandoned by the elite, and the citizenry find themselves down on their backs.

The democratic process may continue to govern the affairs of the nation-state, but the power and resources of the nation-state are being radically constrained, democracy is being rendered thereby irrelevant, and global power is thus being shifted from democratic institutions to elite institutions. Democracy is less and less society's sovereign, even though public rhetoric continues as usual. The deliberations of the commissions go largely unreported: the globalist revolution, profound as it is, is mostly a stealth affair.

According to this analysis, democracy is in considerable trouble indeed, and, by comparison, the future of cyberspace would seem to be a secondary concern. The plot continues to thicken, however, as we proceed to an examination of propaganda and its institutionalised role in the machinery of modern democracy.

Propaganda and democracy

Ownership of media, as a means to influence public opinion and ultimately the policies of government, has always been used to advantage by the economic elite in democracies in the ongoing see-saw struggle for power. Popular movements have also made effective use of the media, from time to time, but in today's increasingly concentrated media industry, elite control over public opinion is for all intents and purposes total. It is so total, in fact, that just as a fish is not aware of the water through which it swims, one sometimes forgets how constrained the scope of public debate has become.

Madison Avenue techniques applied to campaigns, including focus on sound-bites, turn political campaigns into little more than advertising episodes, much like the release of a new toothpaste or hairspray. This has long characterised the situation in the US, and with Blair's takeover of the Labour Party, we've seen the same paradigm imported to the UK.

Even opposition to the status quo is channelled and deflected by media emphasis, as with the militia movements (and Perot and Buchanan candidacies) in the US and the National Front movements in UK and France, which are exploited so as to define anti-globalist sentiment as being reactionary, ultra-nationalist, luddite and racist; similarly, environmental sentiments are regularly interpreted as being anti-Labour, anti-prosperity, 'elitist', etc.

Demonisation of governments and politicians, i.e. blaming government for the problems caused by globalism and excessive corporate influence, is perhaps the single most potent *coup* of the mind-control media in promoting the decline of democratic institutions and the rise of globalism.

Globalisation itself further exemplifies the potency of media propaganda. The rhetoric of neo-liberalism, with its 'reforms' and 'market forces' and 'smaller government', is not just a position within the scope of public debate, but has come to be the very frame of debate. Politicians and government leaders rarely debate whether to embrace globalisation, but compete instead to espouse national policies that best accommodate the demands of globalisation.

As media itself is being globalised and concentrated, it is no surprise that globalisation propaganda is one of its primary products. Whether the vehicle be feature film, network news, advertisement, panel discussion, or sit-com, the presumption of the inevitability of the market forces system and the bankruptcy of existing political arrangements always comes through loud and clear, even when the future's dark side is being portrayed.

The propagandistic success of this barrage is especially amazing in light of the utter bankruptcy of the neo-liberal philosophy itself. The whole experience of the robber-baron era has simply vanished from public memory, in true Orwellian fashion, as we are told that market forces and deregulation are 'modern' efficiencies, the brilliant result of state-of-the-art economic genius.

This historical revision by omission has the consequence that no one brings up the fact that these policies have been tried before and were found sorely wanting – that they led to economic instability, monopolised markets, cyclical depressions, political corruption, worker exploitation and social depravity – and that generations of reform were required to reintroduce competition into markets, to stabilise the financial system, and to institute more equitable employer/employee relations.

The regulatory regimes that were in place before the Reagan–Thatcher era were there for very good reason – they adjudicated, with varying effectiveness, between society's desire for stability and citizen welfare, on the one hand, and the corporate desire for maximising profits, on the other. These regimes implemented a generally reasonable accommodation between the interests of the elite and the people. With the help of today's media propaganda, however, everyone now 'knows' that regulations are nothing more than the counter-productive ego-trips of well- or ill-meaning politico bureaucrats who have nothing better to do than interfere in other people's business.

Again in Orwellian fashion, today's 'reforms' are in fact the dismantlement of reforms – reforms that accomplished the moderation of decades of market forces abuse. The power of the media to define and interpret events, and to set the context in which public discussion is framed, is immense. Old wine can be presented in new vessels, and black can be presented as white, as long as the message is repeated often enough and the facts that don't fit are never given airtime.

The mass media is the front line of corporate globalist control – the very trenches in the battle to maintain elite domination; this fact, in addition to market forces, adds extra urgency to the pace of global media concentration. The central political importance of corporate-dominated mass media to the globalisation process, and to elite control generally, must be kept in mind when attempting to predict the fate of internet culture when commercial cyberspace begins to come online.

In this regard, the treatment of cyberspace and the internet in the massmedia over the past few years lends some portending insights. There are two quite different images that are typically presented, one commercially oriented and the other not.

The first image, frequently presented in fiction or in futuristic documentaries, is about the excitement of cyber adventures, the thrill of virtual reality, and the promise of myriad online enterprises. This commercially oriented image is projected with a positive spin, and suddenly every product and organisation on the block includes a 'www.My.Logo.com' on its packaging and advertising, with in many cases only symbolic utility. Madison Avenue is selling cyberspace – but it is selling the commercial version yet to be implemented, it is pre-establishing a mass market demand.

The other image, very much anchored in today's internet technology, has to do with sinister hackers, wacko bomb conspirators, and luring paedophiles. Those of us who use the net daily find such stories ludicrous and unrepresentative, but because we dismiss such stories we may not realise that for much of the general population, that's all they hear about today's internet. The US CDA (censorship) initiative was fortunately rejected by the US Supreme Court, but the defamation campaign against the non-economic internet continues, in ironic contrast to the boosting images of its commercial future cousin (where no doubt the commercial pornographic offerings will in fact be equally graphic).

The relationship between cyberspace and democracy is a complex one indeed. The internet culture, as the seeming prototype for future cyberspace experience, has enabled a renaissance of open public discussion – a peek at a more open democratic process. This phenomenon has, however, been experienced by a relatively tiny minority of the world's population, and may in fact not survive the commercial onslaught. On the contrary, as a means of universal transport for mass-media products, cyberspace may in fact become the delivery vehicle for even more sophisticated manipulation of public opinion. Rather than the realisation of the democratic dream, cyberspace may turn out instead to be the ultimate Big-Brother nightmare.

In a world where most significant physical and financial events will involve online transactions, and where backdoors are built into encryption algorithms and communications switches, everyone's every move is an open book to those who have the keys to the net nervous system – which would include government agents (on the basis of legality) as well as the operators of the system (on the basis of opportunity and *laissez-faire* non-oversight). From the accounting records alone, there would be a complete trail of almost everything anyone does, and the privacy of this information (from government, police, credit bureaux, advertisers, direct mailers, political strategists, etc.) is far from guaranteed.

Systematic massive surveillance by government agencies would be extremely easy, with the ability to track (undetected) purchases and preferences, financial transactions, physical location, persons and groups communicated with, and the content of communications. There is even the possibility of surreptitious gathering of audio and video signals from home sets that are thought to be 'off' (one up on *1984*), and the remote overriding of home security systems, automobile functions (windows, engine), etc.

In particular, no sizeable group (such as a political organisation or a public-interest group) could exist without having its every deliberation and activity being monitorable by government agencies, depending on how interested the authorities are in its activities.

Mandatory chip-based ID cards or even implants may seem fanciful to many, but the number of government and commercial initiatives in those directions worldwide is cause for serious alarm. Such devices would turn each citizen into an involuntary leaf node of the cyberspace network, his or her chip being remotely monitorable from who knows how many scanning stations, visible or otherwise.

In summary, cyberspace not only promises to be the ultimate commercial delivery channel for the mass-media industry, but its very nature provides the opportunity for the mind-control aspects of the mass media to be carried out with incredible precision, and with full feedback knowledge of who is actually receiving which information, and even what they are saying to their friends about it.

Cyberspace could turn out to be the ideal instrument of power for the elite under globalism – giving precise scientific control over

what gets distributed to whom on a global basis, and full monitoring of everything everyone does (and the accounting records are
always there to go back and follow past trails when desired). Some
readers may find the above scenario far-fetched; they may react with
'It can't happen here'. I would ask them 'What is there to stop it?'.
The corporate domination of societal information flows is an inherent
part of the seemingly unstoppable globalisation process. We turn
now from this 'end view' of the scenario to an examination of how
events are likely to unfold.

Cyberspace: whose utopia?

One can think of digital cyberspace as a kind of utopian realm,
where all communication wishes can be granted. The question is,
who is going to be running this utopian realm? We net users tend
to assume that we'll waltz into this utopia and use it for our creative
purposes, just as we have the internet; but there are others who
have designs on this utopia as well. It is a frontier towards which
more than one set of pioneers have their wagons ready to roll.

Current net users are willing to pay a few cents per hour for their
usage (and complain of any usage charges), and their need for really
high per user bandwidth is yet to be demonstrated. The media
industry, on the other hand, can bring a huge existing traffic onto
cyberspace – a traffic with much higher value-per-transaction than
e-mail and web hits, and a traffic that can gobble up lots of bandwidth. Current users want to pay commodity prices for transport,
whilst the media industry is willing to pay whatever it needs to –
and it can pass on its costs to consumers.

From a purely economic perspective, the interests of the media
industry could be expected to dominate the rules of the road in cyberspace, just as the well-funded land developer can always out-bid the
would-be homesteader. Whether it be purchasing satellite spectrum or
lobbying legislatures, deep pockets tend to get their way.

Economic considerations may not, however, be most decisive in
setting the rules of the cyberspace road: the political angle may be
even more important. Continued mass-media domination of information distribution systems is necessary if the media is to play its
accustomed role as shepherd of public opinion. This role, as we
have seen, is mission-critical to the continuance of the globalisation
process and to elite societal control in general.

It is instructive in this regard to review the history of the radio
industry in 1920s America:

In the 20's there was a battle. Radio was coming along, everyone knew it wasn't a marketable product like shoes. It's gonna be regulated and the question was, who was gonna get hold of it? Well, there were groups, (church groups, labour unions were extremely weak and split then, and some student groups) ... who tried to organise to get radio to become a kind of a public interest phenomenon; but they were just totally smashed. I mean it was completely commercialised.

Chomsky at:
http://www.next.com.au/spyfood/geekgirl/
002manga/chomsky.html)

Other nations followed a different track (note, for example, the BBC in the UK), but this time around it is the US model that is predominating, as we have discussed.

The twin drivers in the commercial monopolisation process are economic necessity (squashing competition from independents for audience attention) and political necessity (maintaining control over public opinion). The mechanisms of domination include concentrated ownership of infrastructure, licensing bureaucracies, information property rights, libel laws, pricing structures, creation of artificial distribution scarcity, and 'public interest' censorship rules. These tactics have all been used and refined throughout the life of electronic media technology, starting with radio, and their use can be expected as part of the cyberspace commercialisation process.

Indeed, the first signs of each of these tactics being deployed are already evident. The US internet backbone has been privatised; consolidation of ownership is beginning in Telecom and in ISP services; WIPO (World Information Property Organisation) is setting down over restrictive global copyright rules, which the US is embellishing with draconian criminal penalties; content restrictions are cropping up all over the world, boosted by ongoing anti-internet propaganda; pricing is being turned over increasingly to 'market forces' (where traditional predatory practices can operate); chilling libel precedents are being set; and moves are afoot to centralise domain-name registration, beginning what appears to be a slippery slide towards ISP licensing ... and these are still very early days in the commercialisation process.

Consider the US Telecom Reform Bill of 1996. Theoretically, it is supposed to lead to 'increased competition' – but what does that mean? There is a transition period, during which a determination must be reached that 'competition is occurring'. After that, it becomes a more or less *laissez-faire* ball game, especially given the ongoing climate of deregulation and lack of anti-trust enforcement. There is no going back, no guarantee that if competition fades, regulation will be restored.

Consolidation is permitted both horizontally and vertically – a telecommunications provider can expand its territory, and it can be sold/merged with content (media) companies. Prices and the definition of services are to be determined by 'the market'. It is as well to keep in mind that the Telecom Bill was pushed through by efforts of telecom and media majors, and well to interpret 'increased competition' in that light. It is also well to keep in mind that the globalisation process tends to propagate the US media model.

Just as the media industry is already becoming increasingly vertically integrated (owning its own distribution infrastructure – satellites, cables, and the like), so the media industry will seek mergers and acquisitions in the telecom industry as the digital network gets closer to implementation.

The ultimate direction is for a single media-communications mega-industry, dominated by a clique of vertically integrated majors, following awesome merger wars among huge conglomerates. Regulation will indeed govern cyberspace but, in accordance with the globalist paradigm, it will be regulation by and for the cartel of majors, as we see presaged by the following recent announcement:

> BRUSSELS (Reuter) – The European Union's top telecommunications official called Monday for an international charter to regulate the internet and other electronic networks. 'Its role would not be to impose detailed rules, except in particular circumstances (child pornography, terrorist networks),' he said. The charter would recognise existing pacts negotiated within the World Trade Organisation and World Intellectual Property Organisation and draw on principles agreed by other bodies such as the Group of Seven top industrial countries, he said.

From an economic point of view, the whole point of monopolisation is to create an 'all the traffic will bear' marketplace – where products are priced on the basis of 'How much will the mass consumer pay for this product?', without a need to consider underpricing competing products. This is the market paradigm that operates today, for example, in cinemas and in video rentals. Films compete there on the basis of consumer interest, not on the basis of price. Copyrights are the foundation of this regime, and WIPO is busily implementing an industrial-grade version of copyright for cyberspace.

Majors will compete with one another, but their competition will be in the realms of content acquisition – seeking to have the most successful product offerings – and coverage – seeking to extend their market territories. Consumers benefit because this competition brings them ever more titillating entertainments, but as citizens they are poorly served because the scope and 'message' of their entertainments (and information) is limited and moulded by corporate interests.

WIPO's strict copyright laws basically mean that each consumer must pay for delivery of each and every media product; it will be illegal to save a copy (on disk or tape) or to forward a copy to someone else, and there will be mechanisms (including technical provisions and surveillance of communications) to provide effective enforcement.

The regulations being laid down for libel, copyright and pornography combine to make internet culture ultimately untenable. A bulletin board, for example, could not be run in open mode – there would need to be, in essence, a bonded professional staff to filter out submissions to avoid liability to prosecution. List owners would be forced to become censors, and to verify contributors' statements, as do newspaper editors. The open non-economic universe of today's internet seems destined to be marginalised just like America's CB-radio or public-interest broadcasting, thus completing the commercial domination of cyberspace and the corporate domination of society.

The power of monopolised ownership, in a *laissez-faire* environment, translates into the power to define service categories, and to set prices according to whatever goals, economic or political, the owners may have in mind.

The ability to distribute media products at reasonable rates to large (but not quite mass) audiences translates into the ability to start up a competing media company – a new film label let's say – with only production costs standing as the major capitalisation required. This is exactly the kind of situation that media cartels wish to avoid; discouraging distribution start-ups is what 'control over distribution' is all about. In the case of television, scarce bandwidth translated into expensive licences and the cartel was easy to maintain.

In the case of cyberspace, the cartel can maintain its traditional distribution-control by defining services, and setting prices, in such a way that media-distribution is artificially expensive, and becomes cost-effective only on a massive scale – requiring massive distribution capitalisation.

In the case of non-commercial group networking, we're talking about small distribution lists, say less than 1,000. What do you think it will cost you to send a message to one person in commercial cyberspace? My guess is that the 'traffic will bear' about as much for a one-page message as for a first-class letter. This may seem overpriced to you, but so what? I consider my voice phone service (and CDs) to be overpriced, but *c'est la vie* in the world of monopoly market forces. The advertising brochure will still be able to boast 'Get your message instantly to anyone in the world – all for one flat rate less than a domestic postage stamp.'

At 25 cents/recipient, say, you can see what happens to the internet mailing-list phenomenon: a 500-person list carries a $125 posting fee direct from the poster to the telecommunications provider. You can play with the numbers, talk about receiver-pays, and point out that corporate users will insist on affordable networking, but it should be clear nonetheless that monopoly-controlled pricing has the power totally to wrench the foundations out from under internet usage patterns. We could soon be back in the days when groups and small publications struggled to scratch together postage for their monthly missives.

The 'media-com' industry will make plenty of money out of one-to-one e-mail messaging, and plenty of money out of their own commercial products. Whether or not they want to encourage widespread citizen networking is entirely up to them – according to their own sovereign cost/benefit analysis. If they don't favour it, it won't happen – except in the same marginalised way that HAM radio operates (only for people with extra time and money on their hands – talking to each other mostly about HAM radio).

One can presume that there will be some kind of commercial chat-room/ discussion-group industry, and one can imagine it being monopolised by online versions of talk radio shows, presided over perhaps by an Oprah Winfrey, a Ted Koppel or a Larry King – with inset screens for 'randomly selected' guests. 'Online discussion' can thus be turned into a new kind of media product, and its distribution economics can be structured to favour the cartel.

The prospects seem dim for both democracy and cyberspace, and cyberspace itself seems to be more a part of the problem than a part of the solution, as with many previous technologies. I will endeavour to address the question of 'What can we do about it?', but first let us revisit the central theme of this collection: 'electronic democracy'.

Electronic democracy: dream or nightmare?

'Electronic democracy' has no generally agreed upon definition – the term is used to refer to everything from community networking and online discussion of issues, to e-mail lobbying of elected representatives. What I'd like to discuss here is one of the more radical definitions of the term: the use of electronic networking to bring about a more direct form of democracy, to short-circuit the representative process and look more to net-supported plebiscites and 'official' online debates in deciding issues of government policy.

There are well-meaning groups on the internet actively articulating and promoting such radical schemes, and to many netizens this kind of 'direct democracy' may seem very appealing (see, for example, Chapter 11). It holds out the promise of cutting through the bureaucratic red tape, reducing the role of corrupt politicians and special interests, and allowing the will of the people to be expressed. In short, it would appear to institutionalise the more promising aspects of internet culture for the benefit of mankind and the furtherance of democratic ideals.

Into this Pollyannic perspective I must, however, cast a dose of realism. Just as it would be naïve to assume that idyllic visions of a global-village commons are likely to characterise commercialised cyberspace, so it would be equally naïve to assume that electronic direct democracy, if implemented, would turn out to be anything like the idealistic visions of its well-meaning proponents.

In examining the future prospects for cyberspace, what turned out to be determinative, at least by my analysis, were the interests of the major players who stand to be most affected by the economic and political opportunities presented by digital networking. It may be the internet community that is the most aware and articulate about cyberspace issues, but they are not the ones who own the infrastructure or make the policy decisions. Similarly, when examining the prospects for electronic democracy, it is absolutely essential to consider the interests of those major players – including corporations, societal elites and government itself – who would be directly affected by any changes made in governmental systems.

If official changes are made to our systems, it is governments who will make those changes – the same governments who are currently presiding over the dismantlement of their own infrastructures and systematically selling out national sovereignty to corporate globalism.

The plain fact is that direct electronic democracy is very much a two-edged sword. Depending on the implementation details – and the devil is indeed in the details – it could lead either to popular sovereignty or to populist manipulation. It could give voice to the common man and woman, or it could be the vehicle for implementing policies so ill-advised that even existing corrupt governments shy away from them – and in such a way that no one is accountable for the consequences.

Consider some of the issues involved: Who decides which questions are raised for a vote? Who decides what viewpoints are presented for consideration? Who decides when sufficient discussion has taken place? Who verifies that the announced tally is in fact accurate? Who checks for vote-adjusting viruses in the software, and who supplies that software?

I do not deny that a beneficent system could be designed, but I don't see how such a system could be reliably guaranteed as the outcome. Even with our current internet and its open culture, the above issues would not be easy to resolve in a satisfactory way. In the context of a commercialised cyberspace, the prospects would be even less favourable.

Let's look for a moment at a direct-democracy precedent. In California, there has long been an initiative and referendum process, and it is much used. This particular system was set up in a fairly reasonable way, and in many cases decent results have been obtained. On the other hand, there have been cases where corporate interests have used the initiative process (with the help of intensive advertising campaigns) to get measures approved that were blatantly unsound, and that the legislature had been sensible enough not to pursue.

In today's political climate, with elite corporate interests firmly in control of most Western governments, the prospects for any radical changes being implemented in a way that actually serves popular interests are very slim indeed. The simple truth is that those interests currently in the ascendancy would be blind fools to allow system changes that seriously threatened the control over the political process that they now enjoy.

If 'electronic democracy' were to be implemented in today's political environment, one can only shudder at how it would be set up, and to what ends it would be employed. The rhetoric surrounding its implementation would, of course, be very attractive – direct expression of popular will, cutting out the corrupt politicos, etc. – but rhetoric is rhetoric, and the reality is something else again, as has become apparent with globalisation itself, or with the US Telecom Reform Bill.

The most likely scenario, in my view, would include a biased statement of the issues, a constrained set of articulated alternatives, and a selected panel of 'experts' who pose no threat to established interests. It would be a show more than a debate – reminiscent of what has happened to public-broadcasting panel shows in the US today, where the majority of panel experts typically 'happen' to come from right-wing think tanks.

Especially disturbing is the intrinsic unaccountability of this kind of direct-democracy process. If an emotionally charged show/debate convinces people to vote for nuking Libya, or expelling immigrants, or sterilising single mothers, for example, no one is afterwards accountable – it was 'the people's will'. The political process is reduced to stimulus–response: a Madison-Avenue-engineered show provides the stimulus, and spur-of-the-moment emotion provides the response.

The history of populism in the latter half of the twentieth century is not particularly promising. Mussolini and Hitler both came to power partly through populist appeals to cut through bureaucracy and bring 'decisiveness' to government. I'd say extreme caution is indicated as regards electronic democracy or any other constitution-level changes at this time of elite ascendancy.

'Electronic democracy', like cyberspace itself, threatens under existing circumstances only to compound the problems faced by democracy. In conclusion, allow me to offer my thoughts on how a democracy-favouring citizenry might best respond to the onslaught of corporate globalisation generally, and how they might approach communications policy in particular.

Democracy and cyberspace: strategic recommendations

Pursuant to the goal of improving the quality of our democracies, it seems to me, upon consideration, that the only effective strategy is an old-fashioned one: grass-roots political organising, creation of broad coalition movements, formulation of common political agendas, and the energetic support of sound candidates, with the objective of rebalancing the elite–people see-saw.

In order to restore balance, national sovereignty must be reinstated over economic and social policies, returning to democracy its potency. Coercively and deceptively imposed debt burdens must be forgiven, and corporations must be effectively encouraged by regulation to be good citizens, just as people are so encouraged by laws. *Laissez-faire* deregulation is just a another name for lawlessness, and gang rule is the inevitable structural outcome, as history – unreconstructed – conclusively demonstrates.

If popular ascendancy can be achieved in this way, then there are all kinds of improvements that could be made to our electoral systems, and increased direct voting might be one of them. Such a popular resurgence would, of course, be an incredibly formidable undertaking, but can we honestly expect significant societal improvement by any other means? In the meantime, novel proposals for system-level changes, even the best intentioned, will be implemented only after being reformulated by the current establishment, to our peril.

Pursuant to the goal of preventing the kind of commercialised cyberspace that has been described above, my recommendation remains the same: broad-based, popular, political activism. The only way in which favourable policies can be expected regarding communications, mass media, excessive corporate influence – or anything else for that matter – is for better candidates and parties to be put in power in the context of a sound, progressive agenda.

Nonetheless, permit me to offer some specific strategic recommendations regarding media and telecommunications policy. The worst aspects of commercialised cyberspace, according to my analysis, arise from monopoly concentration. The indicated policy strategy would be to focus on preventing monopolisation, both the horizontal and vertical variety. To be sure, there are the issues of copyright, censorship and others, but I believe that those are, relatively speaking, already well understood – the problem is simply to gain some influence over them. The monopoly issue, however, deserves a few more words.

Preventing horizontal monopolies is a matter of insuring that competition exists in each market, and setting limits on the number of markets a single operator can enter. Accomplishing this is not rocket science and has been done successfully before. In fact, recent 'reforms', in the case of the US, have largely amounted to undoing not-that-bad regulation. Alternatively, one could specifically sanction horizontal monopolies (as with the classic US RBOC's or pre-privatisation BT), and instead implement regulation that insures sound operation, and same-price-to-all ('common carrier') operation.

Preventing vertical monopolies is a matter of defining 'layers' of service, and preventing cross-ownership across layers. If content owners (media companies), for example, are not allowed to own transport facilities, and transport must be marketed on a same-price-to-all basis, then there would be considerable hope of preserving open discourse in cyberspace. Independent operators (e.g. ISPs) could then afford, and be permitted, to interconnect to the network and offer affordable services to 'the rest of us', as with the internet today.

Part II
Digital democracy and the state

4 Electronic government: more than just a 'good thing'? A question of 'ACCESS'

Eileen Milner

The 'problem' of electronic government

As politicians increasingly identify themselves with what has become euphemistically known as the 'third way', issues around the concept of 'electronic government' have become important and latterly visible on the policy agendas of many major democracies, including Australia, the United Kingdom and the United States. These issues should be viewed as important socially, politically and economically, because they are fundamentally linked to the achievement of the re-engineering of public services in alignment with the twin goals of leveraging both efficiency and effectiveness whilst increasing citizen satisfaction. Yet, seemingly perversely, the general consensus, and in the absence of any informed debate, would appear to be that electronic government is unquestionably accepted as a 'good thing'. The result of this apparent lack of discernible political or public contentiousness has been what can best be described as a tide of 'pilot-mania', where, in countries across the globe, significant resources can be observed in use in relatively small-scale projects, with end results that fail, almost always, to deliver adequate social, economic or political returns in respect of enhanced efficiency or effectiveness of public services.

This chapter points to what the research team at the University of North London perceives as an ongoing imperative to achieve a significant national (and in some cases, such as the European Union, trans-national) focus on working towards the achievement of a coherent and inclusive vision for harnessing information and communications technology (ICT) applications in the re-engineering of public services. If this focus is not achieved, it is argued that, based upon the qualitative research so far carried out, there is every likelihood that 'electronic government' will become a term synonymous with waste: wasted resources and wasted opportunities.

The clear and coherent vision for electronic government that I have alluded to can be achieved only by undertaking rigorous audit and evaluation of existing practices, including the ubiquitous pilot studies that have proliferated in recent years. The data gathered under the auspices of the research discussed here highlights the lack of priority given to pre- or post-implementation evaluation of such pilots. Still more importantly, it requires an acknowledgement amongst senior policy makers that there is a need for informed and 'joined-up' decision making, something that has often been marked by its absence from this particular arena. For example, it may appear somewhat ludicrous that even in the late 1990s, government employees in the UK were unable to e-mail one another or to use internal telephone systems due to the plethora of non-compatible systems that had been purchased over the previous decade. Recognition of these two key inputs to the achievement of meaningful and effective modes of electronic government have given particular focus to the research undertaken at the University of North London. Operating under the acronym 'ACCESS', it has as its underpinning mission the goal of raising senior-level awareness of the opportunities for redefining public sector service design and delivery through the effective use of ICTs.

The term 'ACCESS' has been deliberately chosen for its resonance, particularly in respect of demonstrating its alignment with the issues of social inclusion and exclusion that form a central part of much modern political rhetoric. The research 'brand' also serves as an acronym that is intended to explain more fully the scope of the work undertaken, whereby 'ACCESS' is taken to represent 'A Citizen-Centric Evaluation of electronic government Systems and Services'. The term 'citizen-centric' is used advisedly and, it must be said, with some considerable degree of latitude in respect of precise dictionary definition. It is taken here, for research purposes, to encompass not only the interests, needs, experiences and expectations of the private citizen as an end-user and contributor to the funding of public services, but also the views of other key stakeholding groups, including 'internal' clients of public sector organisations, as well as other groups drawn from the commercial and voluntary sectors. The development of a stakeholder-driven focus on the importance of evaluation strategies and methods is thus suggested as potentially being capable of making a critical contribution to the achievement of appropriate and effective changes to the way in which the public sector organises itself to 'do business'.

The potential for ICTs in public governance

It is important further to contextualise this work by outlining the role and potential contribution that it envisages that ever more powerful ICTs should be capable of making to the process of public governance and service delivery. Examination of the not inconsiderable literature and rhetoric emanating directly and indirectly from the ICT industries, leaves one in little doubt that such organisations wish to be perceived as driving the creation of a bright and exciting new world, where consumers and users of technologies have more choice than ever before. There is also, undoubtedly, much more competition than ever before, both for consumers' 'business' and for their time. Taking the academic perspective provided by the disciplines of Information and Knowledge Management, which underpin the ACCESS research and which firmly position the role of ICTs as an *enabling* one in support of the development of an information and knowledge creating and sharing organisational culture, however, it is possible to hypothesise that the reality can be somewhat harsher, and that the information industry, by its very existence and huge exponential growth, is serving fundamentally to impact upon and dictate the direction of change in society in ways in which few policy makers have actually grasped. In fact, the technology-driven changes that are beginning to emerge, such as the potential for widespread electronic commerce enabled through smartcard and internet applications, as well as the apparently ceaseless flow of innovations enabled by technology more generally, mean that there is an imperative for politicians to acknowledge the fact that we are facing a period of change, the impact of which on society is likely to be more profound than anything we have witnessed since the Industrial Revolution. Lessons from social history leave us in no doubt that when such a period of fundamental structural change takes place, there are inevitably going to be winners and losers. The ultimate and costly irony could well be that issues of social exclusion could, in reality, be exacerbated rather than alleviated as a result of unco-ordinated and poorly focused investments in the achievement of electronic government.

In respect of public governance concerns, it is not enough simply to pay lip-service to the issue of 'losers', or indeed to the potential for disenfranchisement that may be represented through inequitable access to services. Instead, there is a need for a considered approach to focusing upon ways in which ICTs can help to overcome rather than exacerbate issues of access to publicly funded services. The

Australian government has, since 1995, been following a policy agenda in respect of ICT applications in public service that bears some examination in respect of harnessing ICT applications to overcome issues of exclusion. Although very firmly driven by an emphasis upon leveraging the economic performance of public services, innovative usage of technology to break down traditional departmental barriers and therefore simplify citizen access to both information and services has led, the ACCESS team found, to enhanced levels of citizen satisfaction with the performance of services.

Interestingly, Richard Lievesey-Howarth of ICL, although of course clearly identified with the ICT industry, has made a number of important and perceptive observations on the responsibility that both commercial sector providers and public sector organisations and policy makers must accept:

> There is a real possibility that we will create a society of technology 'haves' and 'have nots'. We can disenfranchise millions of people, in fact some will argue that we are in the process of doing just that ... so much is changing ... we must not think of computer-literate people but people-literate computers. The information society can be built around the citizen, rather than the current trend of government building infrastructure around itself. I am talking about a citizen-direct approach, not a government-direct approach. This is a community issue, not a technology issue. We need leaders to tell industry what is good and what is bad. Regrettably there are few leaders doing this.
> (Lievesey-Howarth 1997: 32–3)

The challenge outlined by Lievesey-Howarth is an important one: to set an agenda for the re-engineering of public services that has an inclusive, community-oriented focus. How ironic it is that it is left to an ICT vendor to point to the critical lack of leadership and strategic steer that is evident amongst politicians and senior public service employees in respect of the achievement of change in this area.

The need for leadership

The need for informed and charismatic leadership is clear if the 'disenfranchisement of millions' (Lievesey-Howarth 1997: 32) is to be avoided. The imperative to attain this sense of leadership is paramount, in part at least because of the difficulty of actually engaging informed private citizen input into the design and specification stages of service re-engineering processes. For, as the ACCESS research has established in a global review of practice (enabled particularly by sight of normally confidential opinion and market-research data commissioned by both governments and ICT vendors), end-users are almost always constrained in their ability to imagine alternative and enhanced modes of delivery, by the mental parameters set by their present and past experiences. Asking citizens to adopt an open and creative system of thought in respect of how they might actually like their public services to be designed for use is, it can be argued, at the present time, in practice an almost impossible and marginal value activity. In order to gain any reliable data to lend credibility to changing strategies or new products, governments and vendors alike, when consulting with end-users, almost always resort to using what are essentially 'loaded' questions, where alternative modes of delivery are suggested to participants. This inherently flawed methodology has tended to result in the evaluation of only what is presently available, rather than actually working towards the achievement of the critical breakthrough into analysis of what the citizen actually *needs, wants* and *expects*. What has resulted, has been the plethora of pilots and unco-ordinated projects, the real social and economic value of which must be questioned in the absence of rigorous critical evaluation of outcomes.

The research dichotomy identified here – that between the need to focus up the citizen, whilst at the same time acknowledging the difficulty that the individual is likely to have in conceptualising service delivery methodologies that are free from existing mind-sets and perceptions is an interesting and challenging one. Scenario-based strategies, whereby participants are guided through their perception of an 'event', for example a benefit claim, may provide an interesting and indeed profitable way forward. Such a methodology is undoubtedly resource intensive, however, and it is posited that the current structured questionnaire and interview methodologies in use are likely to prevail until such time as a sufficient body of research can convince policy makers of the economic and value-added rationale for pursuing a scenario-based approach.

Electronic government: the reality

A critical review by the ACCESS team of initiatives and pilots emerging in Europe, North America, Australia and Southeast Asia, served to identify a predominant model in respect of public sector deployment of ICTs in service delivery in the late 1990s. Despite the fact that it is often surrounded by ambitious and persuasive rhetoric, primarily emerging, it must be said, from politicians in all tiers of government, the model is focused almost entirely upon utilising technology to leverage bottom-line performance in terms of achieving cost-savings, often by reducing the level of staffing infrastructure associated with service maintenance and delivery. It is a helpful analogy to think of this model of operation as being represented by a single line of traffic, theoretically moving forward to the inexorable achievement of its identified destination. What it critically does not take account of, however, is that technology does not, indeed cannot, on its own, represent solutions to the complex challenges represented by public service delivery. The reality, our research would suggest, is that the present drivers underpinning developments in this area – politicians' desire for 'improved' services, delivered at reduced or static costs – are fatally flawed in application at least, if not entirely in concept. The single flow of traffic paradigm becomes, then, problematic: with no exits available when problems arise, no ability to vary speed as desired and appropriate and no ability to overtake, then it must be said that 'accidents' are highly likely to occur and, in their wake, to result in damage to political and ICT credibility.

The 'fatal attraction' of ICTs

In the context then of this single-road paradigm, it is important to question the success that has been achieved through large-scale investment in ICTs. A 1996 MORI research report, looking across all sectors of the economy, concluded that 90 percent of organisational investment in ICTs failed to result in an adequate return on the investment made (MORI 1996). What this research alludes to, and indeed supports, are the indicators emanating from the ACCESS work, which suggest that 'pilot-mania' has resulted in considerable 'wasted' investment in ICT solutions in the public sphere. In short, the question must be asked, has an essentially myopic view of the technology as a 'solution' to problems and as a driver of change in the public sphere, served to hinder 'citizen-direct' or even 'government-direct' service development? We must remember also that in the search for solutions and bottom-line performance enhancement, politicians may often be working within a seemingly paradoxical framework of reference: for they are almost universally committed to reducing or maintaining levels of public expenditure whilst, at the same time, operating to a 'bottom-line' not typically found in the commercial sector, that of gaining and retaining an electoral mandate. To this paradox, Bird contributes an interesting perspective by suggesting that there is a very real problem of policy and decision makers being seduced by the powerful draw of technology: 'Too often they (senior managers and politicians) fall in love with a technological innovation that has no practical use in the real world' (Bird 1996: 79)

What this seductive representation of ICT as solutions potentially adds to the single-track road model of electronic government alluded to previously, is an important dimension of impaired vision on the part of those driving the vehicles. A major challenge is how to effectively overcome this. Many of those who co-operated with the first phase of the ACCESS research, and who retained a degree of operational responsibility in their organisations, put forward the view that this attitude towards technologies was likely to be largely a generational issue and that, over time, senior managers in the public sector were likely to have a much more informed and pragmatic view of actual ICT capabilities, applied within a more coherent strategic framework. Subsequent research data gathered from other sectors, particularly the legal and accountancy professions, however, does indicate that even those attaining senior level positions before the age of 40, rarely exhibit the 'hybrid' skills of management that might be expected if ICTs were to be effectively incorporated across organisational planning and functions, as opposed to operating most usually as an entirely separate organisational unit (Milner 1997).

So what does good practice look like?

Having identified the problems associated with current practices in electronic government as arising, primarily, from approaches that closely resemble a single-track road, it is only proper to consider what a model of good practice might look like in terms of necessary inputs and desired outcomes. In the first instance, it is important to take account of what has actually been happening to organisations over the last decade, and to learn from these trends and change factors using a perspective that has been particularly helpful to the formulation of this research:

> The watchwords of the decade are innovation and speed, service and quality. . . . Instead of embedding outdated processes in silicon and software, we should obliterate them and start over.

> We should reengineer our businesses to use the power of modern information technology to radically redesign our business processes in order to achieve dramatic improvements in their performance.
>
> (Hammer 1990: 112)

To 'information technology' we should add the important communications element, for we should not forget particularly the importance of the telephone in redesigning public services; and for 'business' we take the view that you can usefully substitute 'service'; and we have a rationale that actually begins to represent the full potential that the application of technologies offers to the design and delivery of public services appropriate for the twenty-first century. For this to be achieved, the single-track paradigm must be transformed into a three-lane highway, with each lane representing a core area of the model of good practice: citizen involvement and satisfaction; financial performance and employee involvement and satisfaction.

To consider then the first lane of this new highway, it has never been in doubt that importance must be attached to involving and satisfying the citizen (for the purposes of this research regarded as a 'customer' of public services). What has been identified as an area of concern is that this is fundamentally a very difficult process to engage in effectively, particularly at a conceptual level, when you are in practice asking the user to imagine beyond their sphere of experience. There is too little evidence, however, that practice adopted in the commercial sector – whereby a critical part of the development of products/services, particularly those that involve the deployment of technologies, involves extensive attitude and opinion testing – has been carried over with any real commitment or efficacy into the public sphere. Indeed, the ACCESS research revealed that constraints of resources and time meant that, in almost all cases of electronic government initiative considered, inadequate pre-testing took place prior to full-scale launch. This was found to be particularly true when considering the deployment of kiosk technologies, where both the end-user interface and the actual location of the interface, key critical success factors, were inadequately trialled prior to deployment. It is ludicrous that whilst we cannot imagine that a new chocolate bar would be launched without the manufacturer being satisfied, as far as possible, that there was likely to be some degree of market for the product, the same does not appear to hold true for important and expensive developments in public service design and delivery. In this context, the concept of ensuring access to, and time for utilising, 'usability laboratories', where ergonomic and interface aspects of ICTs are tested on potential end-users in carefully monitored situations, is something that should actively be pursued in the public sector. In one instance, a very rare example it must be said, the establishment of such a laboratory by a government department in Astralia, at a cost of some $AU300,000, saved, in its first week of operation, costs of some $AU500,000. This was achieved by identifying, through work with end-users and front-line employees, that the software under test required modifications in order to improve both its operational efficiency and end-user satisfaction with the interface provided.

This emphasis on closely monitoring usability links closely to the second track of the ACCESS highway to success in the electronic government arena, which is to focus on the financial performance of public services. Instead of adopting an entirely bottom-line driven view, however, it is important to acknowledge that some of the greatest potential for achieving cost rationalisation arises from acknowledging and pursuing the potential, enabled by appropriate deployment of ICTs, for facilitating cross-functional methods of working, for reducing duplication of effort and for enhancing the quality of end-user service experience by so doing. This would go some way towards satisfying the 'political bottom-line' alluded to previously, which has much to do with enhancing the public perception of the individual politician or political party responsible for service realignment. An example of such innovative practice is that which is now found in many American states where, in response to alarm at the fall off in voter registration, experiments have been conducted that allow individuals registering their motor vehicles to allow the data used in that transaction to be used to ensure that they are registered as electors. The results of trials using this methodology have been overwhelmingly positive. They have delivered citizen satisfaction with a simplified data-gathering process, alongside the achievement of 'political' goals to increase the numbers of registered voters at significantly reduced unit costs from those achieved by previous initiatives. When viewed in this way, instead of the focus on financial performance operating in what has been a largely negative manner, it becomes embedded in a focused methodology for moving forward the way in which government is structured to 'do business'.

The final strand of the highway put forward here as an exemplar of what needs to underpin the achievement of effective electronic government, is that of focusing upon the important role that public service employees can play in achieving the attainment of service re-engineering. During almost two decades of unprecedented public sector reform, it is perhaps this element of the public service equation that has experienced the greatest stresses resulting from ongoing change processes. In short, the fundamental value of public service employees as organisational knowledge assets and gate keepers has gone unrecognised. By incorporating all levels of staff, particularly those involved in citizen contact, in the redesign of services, especially looking at access and delivery mechanisms, the prospects for achieving positive and sustained change processes are likely to be considerably enhanced. A recognition of the potentially pivotal role of public service employees in contributing to the re-engineering of services has come in 1998 from the British government's newly appointed Minister for Public Service, who has convened a policy group to consider ways in which aspects of Knowledge Management, dependent as it is upon engendering a culture of cross-structural sharing of both explicit and tacit knowledge amongst all levels of employees, can be successfully harnessed.

Conclusion

Perhaps the central message emerging from the research discussed here, and certainly one that should be considered of importance by anyone interested in the issues represented under the label of 'electronic government', is that of the critical importance of gaining and maintaining the attention of political and public service opinion leaders and decision makers. There is too little evidence that this critical group of people have actually grasped the scope and scale of the value that can accrue from approaching the deployment of technologies in a far more considered and integrated manner than has been the case to date. The ACCESS research and model discussed here is, at first acquaintance, a simple one. Yet it demands that those who may seek to apply it acknowledge the scope of the undertaking that it represents. Failure to take account of the underpinning concepts introduced here is likely to result in large-scale waste of scarce resources and, potentially, a missed opportunity to engage the citizen in a more positive interaction and relationship with the services that they resource and mandate through the democratic process.

5 Tools of governance

Elisabeth Richard

The vision of leaders and their governments actively working in collaboration with citizens and interest groups towards measurable goals is prominent in internet-related discourse. This ideal may come from the fact that the internet blends tools for public participation and representation in a unique way. The medium is like a library, a news wire, a deliberation room and a voting booth, all meshed together in a dynamic process at the tip of the citizen's fingers.

The internet's technical architecture also inspires this fantasy. The technological architecture of the internet – a labyrinth of links and nodes, where each new connection brings more strength to the network – is increasingly seen to parallel the emerging relationship between the state and the citizens. The citizen is not only a consumer in the product and service delivery chain, but also a partner in the governance process, a node in this network of lateral connections, which is the model for a healthy civil society.

Much is said about the virtues of electronic democracy, but a technical utopia cannot be reached without the establishment of proper response mechanisms within government. Before the information highway can be used to harness the general public's opinion in a dynamic policy development process, many questions must be addressed. The internet creates a convergence that redefines traditional tools of communication, consultation and decision making, forcing public servants to rethink their roles and the processes and structures designed in the post-war era.

This convergence was evident at the inauguration of the Government of Canada Primary Internet Site. Designed to be the single-window to Canadian federal departments and services, the Canada Site was instantly used just as much as a front door to the government of Canada. Launched a month after a referendum that nearly resulted in the break-up of the country, the site was adopted by

Canadians eager to express their opinions and emotions. Whilst Canada's federal government strategy was primarily to disseminate information through the internet, expectations from the public have forced the federal government to think of their internet presence as a tool for two-way communication with citizens.

After decades of growing disenchantment about public participation in policy development and the democratic process, the public perceives the internet and new technologies as a key element in making deliberative democracies work better. This chapter examines the issues that the Government of Canada Primary Internet Site and federal departments face as they integrate the internet in their strategies, as they try to turn this emerging mass medium into a tool for the community, a potential engine for efficient statecraft.

A confusing convergence

As an expert information management tool, the internet blends most traditional ways of communicating with citizens. Public servants trying to adapt have many models to which to refer: like a news wire, the internet provides easy, quick, updated information; like television or a quality colour publication, it allows the presentation of information in an attractive format; and like a library, it gives access to detailed information upon request. With the same keys on the keyboard, the medium can be used as a tool for deliberation and voting. The monitor offers the same mechanisms as our parliamentary democracy: questions, debate and the vote.

Finally, the internet provides a forum for consultation. The internet allows governments to conduct them in a complete, immediate way, where traditional consultations would use different means. For a specific form of consultation, the public can easily access the documentation put forward by government. The medium allows one to learn by browsing or searching. Discussions can take place, fact sheets can be published, browsed or searched if more information is needed. Opinions can then be recorded.

Virtual public judgement

This potential evokes an online version of the deliberative polling model described by James Fishkin (Fishkin 1991). The process of preparation, documentation, education, deliberation, voting, first round, second round, analysis and so on, can happen on our monitors in front of our very eyes. It can support many of the steps that lead the citizens to become not only voters – and consumers of public services – but also partners of their governments: providing information, reporting back to the citizens, structured consultations and deliberation.

With its unique features as an environment for many-to-many communication, the internet gets automatically associated with this vision. It has the interactivity that facilitates deliberation, the distributed structure that facilitates access and virtuality that reduces constraints of time and space.

Crippled models

The definition of the citizen as a user of public services or as a partner of government has an impact on information policies. These two roles imply different emphases on marketing, information access and consultation. The convergence of marketing, access and consultation tools into one environment exacerbates the confusion. Old models seem incomplete, yet the new model is still undefined. This leads departments to overlook or be confused by many opportunities of the medium.

Information management, for example, is paralysed by a mix of system architecture problems and lack of simple processes. Access to documents is made difficult because they are posted without keywords to facilitate searches. News releases are often published without the URL (Uniform Resource Locator) for the document it refers to on the web. Lack of standard practices of information management among departments makes searching for information by subject difficult. Obstacles that prevent accessing information are exacerbated, as the citizen wanting information about pesticides, for example, might have to browse and search across different databases of information located in the many departments that might carry the relevant information.

Online surveying, compared to scientific methods of public opinion gathering, is another difficult area. It is rarely used in government sites because it is unclear where it fits in the public environment analysis model. Many consultation documents are posted without feedback forms or consultation questions, or methods to collate the comments.

The role of public servants is unclear when it comes to dealing with environments created for debate. Officers in the traditional Whitehall model of the public service, the model for the public service of Canada, are expected solely to explain and inform, whilst debate is the responsibility of elected officials. Internet consultations are often conducted without planning for a moderator, defining the role of program managers involved in the issue, or planning a process for a quick response by an elected official. Should there be a moderator, and if so, is the moderation done from the point of view of the minister, the public or the departmental client group?

Planned for one-way communication

Like other Western countries, the main concern for the Canadian federal government in establishing web sites has been to disseminate information. Two-way communication was not part of the original strategy.[1] A survey conducted in the autumn of 1997 by the G7 Government online and the International Council for Information Technology in Government Administration[2] shows that 'dissemination of information is ... considered to be a key motivation which indicates that web sites are primarily considered to be an effective publishing medium'.

In the same survey, by contrast, twelve of the sixteen countries surveyed assigned low importance to establishing web services to acquire information. Even though half the countries reported isolated cases that were documented in some of their departments, there was no evidence to suggest that any central policies for public consultation existed in any of the sixteen countries surveyed.

In an OECD study[3] (Gualtieri forthcoming), Roberto Gualtieri finds that 'traditional instruments are still mainly used to gather information for policy purposes: letters, written submissions, telephone conversations, informal meetings ... and so on. The information and communication technologies are not much used to gather policy information'.

The public wants in

This one-way strategy is limited in the public's view. This was clear as soon as the Government of Canada Primary Internet Site was inaugurated. A wide variety of questions and comments are presented by citizens everyday, with the comments box often mirroring the day's major news headlines.

A recent survey shows that the new Information and Communication Technologies and the internet are perceived by the public to be among the most useful tools to gather the views of Canadians, more useful than townhall meetings or mail-outs (EKOS Research Associates 1998).

As governments are trying to integrate citizens in the decision-making process, traditional communication, consultation and decision-making processes need to be reviewed. According to the OECD study, departments are already struggling with impacts brought upon the decision-making process by the Information Society: a more complex policy-making process and an increasing difficulty in setting and maintain an agenda, which has 'resulted in an enormous stress on marketing policy decisions' (Gualtieri forthcoming).

> Indeed, for a medium that fosters massive talk, tools for massive listening have to be created. As this participant to a UK Collaborative Open Group, one of the first discussion groups fostered by a national government, puts it: The internet for the first time allows for active participation and interaction between the governors and the governed. Mass listening is a hard problem, the number of people wishing to comment on a particular government program will inevitably outstrip the ability of decision-makers to analyse the response.
>
> (Halam-Baker)

Yet, mass listening is an issue that will not go away. In his critique of the Information Society, Daniel Yankelovitch says

> We need to recognise that the true problem is not a lack of information. Rather the problem lies in the tendency of governments to objectify themselves and, in so doing, to distance themselves from ordinary citizens ... The solution is more genuine dialogue, not more information.
>
> (Rosell *et al.* 1995: 249)

Underused tools for mass listening

For governments of the post-war era, opinion polls are the preferred tool for mass listening. It is no surprise that, with off-the-shelf survey and reporting packages available and affordable, web surveys have proliferated. Media sites use them to tally opinions about issues; commercial sites gather information about customer tastes. In contrast, departments have been slow to integrate them in their strategies. They are not sure how they can use them as a listening tool or how they can be designed to feed into the policy development process.

The private sector has been quick to use online surveys in the form of questionnaires, to create databases of information on client profiles and tastes that can be used to customise the services through the web site, and to follow up with further relevant information. They are used to identify market segments and reach out to specific groups (Martin 1996).

Some federal departments are integrating online surveys in their opinion-gathering tactics. They define them more like affordable focus groups, a structured, qualitative summary of e-mail. The Canadian Department of National Defence is planning to conduct regular snapshot surveys using an off-the-shelf survey and reporting package (although formal surveys, polling and focus testing, more methodologically sound data collection and analysis will still be conducted) (Pasian 1998).

Distribute the listening

The private sector has also been quick to set up self-help user groups. The internet brings a new dimension to relationships with the client-group. In a medium where everybody does the talking, self-help user groups are a way to distribute the listening, reduce the resources needed to answer all the requests, and reduce the response time. Product-oriented conferences on the major online services are a good example of this.

Some Canadian federal sites fostered a similar community spirit very early on. For some time, the guest book set up on Health Canada's web site, one of the first Canadian federal departments to encourage participation of Internauts, served as an informal self-help resource. Health practitioners used it as a professional bulletin board, to post conferences and to ask for information.

The department accepted the risk that the bulletin board would be used not only to exchange information but also to debate an issue. Of course, it was only a matter of time before some controversy emerged on the bulletin board. The pasteurised cheese controversy – a recommendation that would have made it difficult to distribute non-pasteurised cheese and that created a lot of public reaction – generated an avalanche of postings. This led to questions about whether this public space was the right vehicle for such a debate and, if it was, whether this called for an official intervention from the department. The decision was to let the debate follow its course, but the question remained.

Virtual communities

Health Canada fostered the creation of Health Net, creating a public space for health practitioners. The Department of Justice also opened a site which was quickly adopted by the community, 'Access to Justice'. The virtual community was helpful in communicating with stakeholders and discussing areas of interest. The web site served as an issue clearinghouse.

By reducing the boundaries between government and stakeholders, the internet also created questions of accountability. The message coming from some community members might be perceived as coming from the host organisation. On the Access to Justice web site, for example, opposing groups on some issues were at one point challenging each other's right to appear on the web site.

Growing pains for underdeveloped models

As the vision of citizen-as-a-partner develops, the increasing use of the internet will encourage new models of governance to emerge, where leaders and their governments work hand in hand towards measurable goals and results. At present, however, we see old models being stretched, pulled and dismantled.

The decision-making model is considerably stretched. The old model of decide–announce–defend is challenged by the emergence of the citizen-as-a-partner. Networking online allows government to work closely with communities of interest. Citizens expect to be part of this dialogue.

Theoretically, this gradual consensus-building approach with citizens-as-partners would reduce the amount of marketing needed after a decision is made. The close ties with interested communities – fostered through web sites and discussion groups – would allow trial balloons to be tested, thereby stretching the public environment analysis over the decision-making process. Initiating an online discussion and creating quick surveys on issues, is a potentially healthier way of coming to public judgement than relying on public opinion polls.

Avalanche of self-identified stakeholders

The internet also potentially allows stakeholders to self-identify, which means the number of stakeholders could multiply. This is a challenge to the present model of consultation with a controlled group of stakeholders. In the absence of thorough information management practices, the collection of comments can turn into a programme manager's nightmare, particularly when the moderation of the discussions is weak (Saad 1997).

Ironically, this cumbersome process is said to turn to the advantage of some public servants. According to the OECD study:

> For decision-makers, the source is rarely the internet but the bureaucrat or other advisor who has culled the internet (and other sources) for information to support the policy proposals under discussion. The bureaucrat does the selecting, ordering and presentation of the information. An undetermined amount of filtering takes place at this stage. The bureaucrat becomes the primary source of information. The internet is secondary. Thus it cannot be assumed that the technologies in the hands of public servants will in and of themselves lead to greater democratic decision-making. On the contrary, the new technologies give middle-level bureaucrats added weight in advising their seniors and tend to shift influence if not power toward their hands.
>
> (Gualtieri forthcoming)

Whether or not they want to engage officially in discussions with their communities of interest, departments cannot escape online monitoring. With commentators like Matt Drudge in the US, who influences public opinion using solely internet mail, public environment analysis is now bound to include newsgroup monitoring, media monitoring and public opinion research as tools for massive listening.

Bridge vs tower

Whilst some departments have used their servers and web sites to strengthen their ties with their communities of interest, some have established the web site and the internet as direct channels to the population. This channel allows them to bypass the media and tell their story directly to the public, a considerable shift for information officers trained to write for the Press Gallery.

With the internet providing a direct channel to the population, departments have a new tool for issues management. The internet becomes a tool to send unfiltered messages to the public, keeping intact the departmental view. Some are toying with the idea of using a version of the 'House cards', the comments prepared for government ministers to respond to the questions in the House of Commons. For web masters trying to provide end-users with a quick, direct, point of view on the departmental issues of interest to them, these cards are seen as the best, most reliable, source, considering that there is no time for information officers to finesse messages that need ten steps of approval. This would represent a considerable change, considering that the House cards are not public documents.

Public enquiries: spectre or gold mine?

In the good old days of gopher sites, computer branches who were managing the sites came up with their best crack at tackling two-way communication: the FAQs. Long lists of answers to Frequently Asked Questions were posted in the hopes that readers would see them before they hit the keyboard with yet one more question. They were designed not to show that someone was listening, but to reduce the volume of e-mails. Considering how they were presented – long lists of answers – the method was more or less a success. No system has yet surfaced to replace the old FAQs.

This is a sharp contrast with the automated databases of frequently asked questions, and various wizards that guide the customers in the private sector, where public enquiries are seen as a gold mine, a tool to build a relationship with the customers. The private sector uses them as information-gathering tools, to find out what customers want and to respond by promoting services. A large array of online tools deals with public enquiries.

In the public sector, the possibility of an e-mail avalanche is omnipresent. In the federal government, answers to public enquiries are seen as a timid information-dissemination technique. Government handling of public enquiries on the internet remains paralysed by the possibility of volume, and therefore few proactive techniques are used. The standard individual e-mail answer, often provided by relatively senior and definitely overburdened programme managers, still prevails. Many programme managers in the Canadian government process over fifty e-mails a day. This might increase when their e-mail addresses become included in the telephone directory, as is planned in the months to come.

Whilst a limited number of Canadian departments are starting to test similar tools, on the Government of Canada Primary Internet Site a reference officer answers all questions and regularly updates the list of FAQs. New FAQs are seen as leads for creating new pages of interest. The Canada Site is also experimenting with a database technology to answer questions.

Comments on the Canada Site are also catalogued by issue. The ease and informality of the internet makes them different to formal mail, although for some correspondence officers they are to be catalogued in the same basket: an involuntary consultation, or in other words, a listening tool.

Dislocated members

With its inherent capacity to create instant coalitions of interest, the web site creates demands for coalitions within the departmental structure. Pressures to co-ordinate information have always been present in government, but the internet exacerbates the need. There is one citizen, in front of one screen, looking for information about one issue. Even though the answer might come from a variety of branches and departments, the citizen expects some homogeneity in the results. The citizen expects all departments or branches to provide co-ordinated information, not just one and not the other. The accessibility of one part of the information makes the absence of the rest even more evident. The public also expects to see a common look and feel to this information. After a decade of decentralisation, the internet is forcing departments to co-ordinate their information and messages. The technology allows government departments to think horizontally, and they are forced to adapt.

Interdepartmental initiatives have responded to this need, but they have had considerable difficulty overcoming the lack of standards and interoperability of many sources of information. Browsing on the web made evident, for example, the variety of logos, and the Canada trademark, central to the federal government identity, seemed to disappear. The need to make information available by subject has exacerbated the information management failures and the difficulty to get departments, branches and individual authors to index their documents in a common way.

Listening tools

A common way of cataloguing interactive applications is to determine whether they allow for many-to-many communication (many speakers, many listeners) or only many-to-one (many speakers, one listener) messages. They are all listening tools. Generally, many-to-one applications require resources, but guarantee control, whilst many-to-many applications, unless they are moderated, are perceived as a riskier platform because they allow end-users to broadcast their thoughts.

Many-to-one applications

Surveys

See above.

One-way guest books

They are an informal, non-directive version of the survey and can be as simple as a form with space for the name, address and other personal information of the user, and an area for comments. Like surveys, they are ideal for creating a database of users.

Frequently asked questions

See above.

Quizzes

Many programs aimed at the young, or those that have a strong educational component, have taken advantages of the quiz format. This web technology, simple to program, allows for instantaneous results – a rewarding feature for the end-user.

Many-to-many applications

Many-to-many applications play a different role, allowing broadcasting from a wide range of sources. This makes them more of a community tool. Tapping into this community can sometimes save resources, but may denote new issues of accountability.

Two-ways guest books

They allow for comments and questions from end-users to be automatically broadcast on the web. Guest books are sometimes used like a Usenet newsgroup, as a forum to exchange resources, or to create a calendar of community events.

Mailing lists

When set for two-way communications, they allow for an e-mail broadcast of comments and questions. Various agencies use them to obtain feedback from stakeholders and to discuss programme issues.

Web-based conferences

Applications have multiplied in the last year, from the simple postings allowing one to follow threads of discussion topics, to library areas and voting components. According to the case studies documented by individual departments, most principles of online conferences apply to consultations on policy issues. A small group of participants with a precise goal have the best chances to obtain meaningful results. Daily summaries of discussions help to create consensus and move the discussion. Careful preparation of the information management processes in order to obtain a solid database of facts and opinions is key. An analysis of a virtual workshop on regulatory efficiency for the minerals and mining industry shows that careful information management was a matter not of cost but of preparation, since many of the technologies are now available off the shelf (Hale and Sourani 1998).

Newsgroups

Simple, cross-platform, easier to access than web-based conferences, they don't clutter the e-mail like list serves; they also don't seem to have been picked up as a government tool. It has been suggested that the controversial nature of newsgroups is what has kept government from using them as a tool. The free debate style of Usenet is identified as too different from the neutrality expected from the machinery of government in a parliamentary democracy. In Canada, a can.announce newsgroup has remained inactive.

Live discussions

Recent developments have made them secure and easy to use. They have been used to create a variety of special events ranging from policy-oriented discussions to questions and answers with rock stars. Moderated live chats are a form of radio open line, which includes the public, the guest and the moderator directing questions. The technology allows questions to be blocked until the moderator has screened them, which protects guests from potentially embarrassing questions.

Conclusion: framework needed for models

Some Canadian departments are among the pioneers of online communications. Whilst no initiative to foster information gathering through the internet has been centrally initiated, as with other G7 countries, many isolated experiences have been attempted in individual departments. Similar questions keep coming up:

- What is the most suitable online discussion framework for a given form of consultation?
- When should it be real-time, or asynchronous?
- What is the role of officials?
- How close are decision makers to the process?
- How do public servants contribute to discussions?
- If the process is iterative, how should programme information be presented in a dynamic way?
- How are unsolicited comments from users processed?
- In what instances is a survey form recommended?
- What are the standards for response time?

Know-how has been accumulated over the years through regional, national and municipal efforts all over the planet, but it is used and documented only in bits and pieces. A clear framework is lacking. How do our hierarchical, horizontal, public service structures fit into this environment of connections that are no longer horizontal, but increasingly lateral and diagonal?

Without new consultation, communication, correspondence and programme management models, citizens cannot expect to become partners in the governance process. Without ensuring that their administrations are adapted to this new environment of links and nodes, governments cannot expect to take an active role in a structure increasingly described as the model for a healthy civil society.

Notes

1 Government of Canada Internet Strategy in the Government of Canada Internet Guide p. 5 http://www.tbs-sct.gc.ca/

2   Government Use of the internet, G7 Governments Online and International Council for Information Technology in Government. P.7. http://www.open.gov.uk/govoline/latest1.htm

3   This study was commissioned by OECD Public Management Services and its contents do not necessarily reflect the views of the governments of OECD member countries.

6 Electronic support of citizen participation in planning processes

Klaus Lenk

Introduction

Discussions concerning opportunities for the support of political debates and decision-making processes through information systems are long standing. The relevant issues have been discussed for at least three decades. Around 1970, the attention focused on comprehensive service arrangements of a so-called 'information utility', which was expected to materialise on an infrastructure of bi-directional TV cable networks. Next to information services and online shopping, the pros and cons of online voting and polling and of supporting democratic participation in planning processes were hotly debated in North America (for a summary of this discussion see Lenk 1976). The merging of data bank and communication technologies that took shape in the late 1960s provided the basis for new concepts. These concepts sought to support democratic decision making by providing relevant information to stakeholders or to the general public and by structuring debates and lines of reasoning. Examples include a system called MINERVA, developed by Amitai Etzioni, which was intended to intensify direct democracy by supporting debates on particular issues. Similar experiments were conducted in Germany by systems scientist Helmut Krauch (Lenk 1976).

Despite a few pilot projects, this early debate was mostly academic. Over the years, it has never ceased completely (van de Donk and Tops 1995), but it is only now that information technology has 'come of age' that wide-ranging applications in the field of citizen participation can be considered seriously. The main characteristic of systems that support local democracy and participation in decision making is a combination of several technological 'ingredients' that are tied together in innovative ways. Among them are not only networks that support communication and give access to information resources, but also systems that make use of the potential of information technology to process information in different ways. Seen from this angle, ICTs can be used as a technology that *organises* information. This property of IT can be used to structure debates so that some of the impediments to stronger democratic participation can be overcome. As an example, more opinions could be taken into account in the decision-making process than would have been possible in a face-to-face meeting that is not supported by adequate technological tools.

This chapter follows some of the lines that were drawn three decades ago – without, however, espousing the optimistic model of man ('venture on more democracy', according to the then German Chancellor Willy Brandt) that underpinned the early discussions about extending citizen participation in planning and decision-making processes.

The potential

Taking our start from the basic 'ingredients', we recognise that information systems can support and promote citizen participation in public planning as well as mediation processes in different ways:

1   by providing information on a problem and its background (including interactive and multimedia forms and 'virtual reality' techniques);
2   by supporting communication processes (including asynchronous modes and communication between spatially distant persons, i.e. 'teleco-operation');
3   by structuring debates;
4   by directly supporting decision processes, e.g. through electronic voting.

Let us consider some of these ingredients in more detail.

Citizen-oriented information systems

Information provision through citizen-oriented information systems is at present making substantial progress. Due to the attraction of the world wide web, and also to the promotion of kiosk systems, various citizen-oriented information systems are now operational. The main functions of these information systems are not yet specifically aimed at democratic decision making. They concern:

- the provision of basic information and referral services ('Where do I get what, and how?');
- the provision of information on eligibility for public services and for money transfers, as well as on legal rights and duties;
- the provision of other information of general interest, including information about planning processes.

(Lenk *et al.* 1990: 100–1)

It took quite some time before the potential of citizen-oriented information systems began to be realised. In particular, the introduction of 'videotex' systems in the early 1980s (the French MINITEL, the German BILDSCHIRMTEXT and the British PRESTEL) was not conducive to the development of useful and acceptable citizen information systems. One reason for this was that the handful of citizen information systems developed on this platform sought to provide information directly to citizens. An alternative approach would have consisted not of making these systems directly available to citizens via a Kiosk or a network, but of empowering contact persons who have a mediating function of assisting individual citizens in their dealings with authorities (Lenk *et al.* 1990). Some German cities, such as Berlin, have developed citizen information systems that try to do both: provide information directly to citzens who have simple questions relating to public services, rights and duties, *and* support street-level contact persons in situations where they are asked by citizens for information.

Whilst such systems are finally gaining ground, they still fall short of delivering information that is of specific use in promoting citizen participation in public decision making. As a counterweight to one-sided administrative reforms that promoted efficiency and effectiveness at the expense of democratic participation, however, we can soon expect a cultural change in favour of providing more information to citizens beyond their consumer roles, in order to help them to participate in public affairs. When we developed reference models for citizen information systems in the late 1980s, we tried to anticipate the provision of what we called 'structural' information, e.g. on planning procedures, on public institutions, and also on proposals for zoning plans etc. (Lenk *et al.* 1990). At that time, neither the cultural dispositions to invest in similar systems nor the required network platforms were present; but a breakthrough seems imminent now.

Support of communication

It is obvious that the perspectives of supporting political communication through internet-based 'free-nets' or the like are tributary to a model of democracy that corresponds to the Athenian agora (Schalken and Tops 1995). Most uses of the internet in connection with enhancing democracy still centre around facilitating a virtual marketplace: they allow an unstructured communication over distance and in an asychronous mode. The philosophy underlying 'free-nets' is one of endless debate that should, following Habermas, be conducive to agreement and consensus (Schalken 1998). Experience with 'digital cities' experiments indicates that there is a disregard of the organisational problems involved in bringing democracy to work where larger numbers of people are concerned and where issues have become extremely complex and policies overlap. This makes participation not very meaningful beyond collecting some opinions about policy or planning proposals. In Germany, draft legislation has been exposed for comment on the internet. The results so far are mixed, and they will hardly improve if the present over-representation of young, male and well-educated participants in such debates does not give way to a more equal distribution. Moreover, if discussion forums do not succeed in structuring the information communicated by the participants, the time needed for gaining access to and participating in the discussions will continue to grow.

Structuring debates through Issue-Based Information Systems

Despite the failure of most local democracy experiments to structure debates and to avoid information overload, the internet provides an infrastructure on which conceptually interesting information systems can be based. The idea of 'Issue-Based Information Systems' (IBIS), developed by Horst Rittel in 1970, was rediscovered in the late 1980s. Such systems can be used to structure debates on controversial issues. Structuring of discussions may also be helpful to promote the discourse among discussants or it may be applied in mediation procedures. The structuring of information is particularly useful in the early stages of the policy process, i.e. for identifying problems and elaborating solutions (Isenmann and Reuter 1996). IBIS proceed from the assumption that not all the knowledge relevant to the issue is available at the beginning of a decision-making process, but that it must first be worked out and stated explicitly

(Isenmann and Reuter 1996: 174). IBIS provide a framework of categories according to which the various contributions to a discussion may be arranged and which makes it possible to recognise the interrelations between these contributions. Contributions to discussions are categorised as questions, answers and arguments raised. Thus a network of problem-related information emerges.

IBIS can therefore be used as a method of structuring communication in problem-solving procedures. This can even be useful after all arguments have been raised, in that all interests can be made transparent for the final decision making. However, as far as citizen participation in planning procedures is concerned, the exploration and structuring of the problem, the identification of a problem and the elaboration of alternative solutions have priority.

Decision Support Systems: a tool for promoting democracy?

Decision Support Systems (DSS) adopt a different approach, since they deal with decision problems in a formal–rational rather than a discursive way (Kraemer and King 1988). Assumptions – no matter how they where arrived at – are analysed and their implications evaluated. Many DSS have been developed in the 1980s; most frequently they were spin-offs from military research. Their approach is a rational one: those variables that (according to the decision makers) have an impact on the ultimate decision are interrelated and rated; subsequently, the results obtained are reviewed. The rationalistic model inspired systems that combine formal and probabilistic methods with forms of visualisation, which help decision makers to apprehend the essentials of a problem. In such a way, counter-intuitive consequences of alternative courses of action can be discovered. No importance is, however, given to the fact that there may be more than one decision maker, and that within a group of decision makers, views may be conflicting.

By contrast, the so-called Group Decision Support Systems (GDSS) explicitly support collaborative processes within a group – e.g. agenda setting, brainstorming, commenting, voting, and documenting the results of deliberations. Groups that use these tools normally rely on a facilitator who structures the debate both from a technical and from a substantive standpoint. The pros and cons of GDSS are now well known (Schwabe 1994): results are obtained faster, but perhaps at the expense of a deeper consensus that would promote the implementation of the results obtained. Some of the well-known shortcomings of meetings and of 'groupthink' may be overcome, in that the opinions of the most vocal people will not be overrated at the expense of others. Also, a skilful facilitator might prevent groups from exhibiting extreme forms of behaviour that their members individually would not have shown; in this way, the greater inclination of groups to take risks and an exaggerated reliance on their power of judgement could be counterbalanced.

Electronic Meeting Rooms are the most important form of GDSS. They are designed to promote decision making in meetings with physically present participants. An Electronic Meeting Room comprises 12–24 work stations. Screens and keyboards that have been sunk into the tabletop make it possible to key in statements while keeping eye-contact with the other members of the discussion group. The results are visualised via a beamer for the whole group. Most widely known is the software GroupSystems V. developed by Jay Nunamaker *et al.* at the University of Arizona. It consists of a number of tools that a facilitator controls by means of an agenda tool. The following activities are supported: brainstorming, categorisation, commenting, voting, designing (whiteboarding), drafting hand-outs, generating protocols (reports), saving results and the personal notes of the participants.

Some public administrative bodies already use such systems for their strategic planning sessions. The Dutch Ministry for Welfare and Public Health and the Amsterdam Police, for instance, use the group decision rooms of the Technical University at Delft. Experience gained in the USA has shown that the use of these systems is particularly apt at promoting the generation of ideas. An experiment conducted at Stuttgart, Germany, is aimed at introducing such systems into local council committees (Krcmar and Schwabe 1995).

Experimental designs

As this short review of the basic building blocks of systems to support local democracy shows, there are many approaches to participation-enhancing information systems that have not yet been tried out. Progress in promoting stronger forms of democracy at the local level is therefore possible. It is also probable that steps in this direction will be undertaken in a climate where administrative reform so far has rather neglected democratic participation, but where a new consumer orientation joins forces with older tendencies to give people a say in decisions immediately concerning their lives.

Innovative systems can therefore be expected in which elements of the potential for the supply of information, for the support of communication and for the support of decision-making processes are combined. The design of comprehensive systems for the support of citizen participation can profit especially from developments in the field of CSCW (Computer-Supported Cooperative Work). Access to information and communication support for the participation of citizens are only a precondition for the efficiency of the approach. The more complex issues in designing such systems arise in structuring debates and allocating rights to raise issues and comment on them. So far only little experience has been gathered regarding the use of such combined systems that support the structuring of decision making beyond the level of information supply (cf. Isenmann and Reuter 1996).

An example of new types of participation-enhancing information systems is provided by the GEOMED project, which is funded by the European Union. It comprises:

- information services: access to geographical information (GIS) in planning procedures;
- documentation services: a 'shared workspace' for the elaboration, storage and retrieval of documents and contributions to the debates of a planning process or a mediation procedure; and
- mediation services: assistance to human mediators of a round table through an IBIS.

A wide variety of planning tasks require access to geographical information, which is typically represented in maps. Thus the accessibility of geographical information in heterogeneous GIS systems over the internet has to be established. GEOMED users are able to access, view and manipulate maps embedded in HTML pages from ordinary www client PCs. Other information present in the www will also be made accessible. The 'shared workspace' provided by the documentation services for storing and retrieving documents and messages related to particular geographical planning projects, provides a convenient way for ordinary users to add information to the hyperspace of documents available.

This approach is being tested currently by the city of Bonn in three planning processes. One of these concerns the high-speed train link between Cologne and Frankfurt. It can be seen as a prototype of an asynchronous process where participants are not located in the same place. Essential to the model is the support through a

CSCW 'shared workspace'. An administrator prepares a GEOMED workspace, making background information available by setting links to basic documents and preparing access to the system for the participants. Of particular importance is the display of maps and other geographic information (GIS viewer). For those participants who prefer to act in the traditional way, the facilitator brings their contributions to the shared workspace. There is an initial set of relevant information, comprising plans together with explanations and statements of the planners. Participants can add their statements and opinions, and they can mark and annotate plans. Planners can respond to these annotations and they may be entitled to modify plans immediately. The Issue-Based Information System facilitates structuring and mediation of the debate.

Democracy at the local level as an organisation problem

Experiments such as the one briefly mentioned here try to find new ways of structuring debates, but efforts have already been made at structuring debates without technological support. It would be particularly interesting to support participative planning processes that have already been structured (Mayer 1997: 88ff.). In particular, this applies to the so-called 'planning cell' developed by Peter Dienel (Dienel 1991). Randomly selected participants are given a paid leave from workday obligations for a limited period of time, in order to work out solutions for given planning problems with the assistance of advisers on procedure. The planning cell method is primarily used for planning decisions involving infrastructure and new technologies. A so-called Citizen Report (Bürgergutachten) is generated that contains suggestions for solutions to political problems. The considerable value of the suggested solutions – e.g. those for the design of the German ISDN – has been widely appreciated.

Depending on their design, information systems embody and represent structures that may help to overcome well-known organisational problems related to democracy: the bringing together of like-minded people, the structuring of debates or the embedding of rules that give a better say to people who have difficulty in expressing themselves. Local democracy, like any democracy involving more than a small group of people ('seven plus/minus two'), is clearly a problem of organisation. Information technologies, beyond their function of supporting telecommunication and providing access to stored information, are technologies of organisation, and it is therefore, important that experiments like those described continue and that we gain a clearer impression of the manifold forms that electronic support of citizen participation could take.

Special attention must be given to the effects that the various systems and a combination of them have on the organisation. The structuring effects of the respective instruments are beyond doubt (Schwabe 1994). In the available group discussion systems, for instance, the facilitator wields considerable power. In general, participants consider his powerful position to be helpful, and therefore accept it. It is not clear, however, whether this also applies to group discussions with a great potential for conflict.

The necessity to develop adequate procedures and to structure participatory decision-making processes is already reflected in a system like the 'planning cell'. Structuring is particularly important to processes in which the voices of different groups of stakeholders should not be given the same weight. One may speak in this context of a 'scaled' round table (Steinmüller 1993).

It is necessary now that innovations in the practice (and also the theory) of democracy and CSCW research should fuse together. Substantial improvements in 'electronic democracy' will not result from a simple orchestration of unstructured participation with some 'tools'. Rather, innovations in the practice of democracy and the development of the potential of 'Groupware' might combine to open up new ways of promoting stronger forms of democracy at the local level. It is thus worthwhile to experiment with new approaches.

7 Developing digital democracy: evidence from Californian municipal web pages

Matthew Hale, Juliet Musso and Christopher Weare

Introduction

This chapter reviews proposed reforms intended to make the American democratic system more participatory, and examines the role that new communications technologies might play in improving democratic participation. In the words of Benjamin Barber, the failure of American democracy has 'become the tedious cliché with which we flaunt our hard pressed modernity' (Barber 1984: xii). Negative political campaigns, undue influence of special interests, and campaign financing scandals suggest that our democratic system is in crisis (Southwell 1986; Dionne 1991; Chen 1992; Ansolabehere 1994). There is little agreement, however, regarding the sources of democratic failure, much less the appropriate means to reform the democratic system. Lack of specificity about the shortcomings of our democratic system has muddled the debate regarding the political effects of new technologies.

To explore how the internet and the world wide web might be used to improve the democratic process, we focus on three types of improvements intended to enhance citizen participation. First, we examine the contention that citizens do not have the civic education necessary to act meaningfully in the political process. From this perspective, technology might provide citizens with better information, elucidate values and contribute to public debate regarding public issues. Second, we consider the perception that there is a generalised apathy towards civic affairs among the general public, and a decline in the 'social capital' required to build political community and encourage participation. The question is how telecommunications technologies might facilitate meaningful group interactions. Third, we discuss the idea that citizens are disconnected from their government. We examine the extent to which technology might bridge the gap between the governing class (elected officials, government workers, the political elite) and ordinary citizens.

We then turn to an analysis of 290 municipal web sites in California to examine whether the design of these new technologies corresponds to our three models of participatory reform. Our conclusions are twofold. First, we suggest that the internet is likely to support only incremental modifications to the democratic system, not the more fundamental changes identified by proponents of democratic revitalisation. Second, we conclude that municipal use of telecommunications technologies concentrates primarily on *information provision*, not the communication linkages that might improve the quality of democratic discourse. These results are particularly discouraging, given that municipal governments are close to the people and have been argued to be the training ground for democracy.

Improving participatory democracy

As use of the internet and world wide web by citizens has increased, a number of scholars have touted the web as a means to increase democratic participation and strengthen political community (Barber 1984; Arterton 1987; Beamish 1995; Bonchek 1995; Grossman 1995; Bimber 1996; Ward 1996). It has been argued, for example, that new information technologies will transform the nature of political activity by infusing American representative democracy with the direct democratic ideals of the Ancient Greek city state (Grossman 1995), or by fostering local communitarian political structures (Bimber 1996). This literature has suffered from a lack of a structured framework for analysing the potential of new technologies to improve participatory democracy, and from a dearth of empirical evidence regarding actual use of technologies.

This chapter examines more systematically whether telecommunications technologies might enhance civic participation by improving information and fostering communication between citizens and public officials at the local level. In this section, we draw from the literature in administrative theory and democratic participation, to identify three major factors that inhibit citizen participation in the political system:

1   inadequate civic education,
2   citizen apathy, and
3   a disconnection between citizens and their representatives.

In the next section, we tie these three factors to potential uses of telecommunications technologies at the municipal level to facilitate citizen participation. We then turn to evidence on the technology implemented in web sites serving California cities, to determine the extent to which current use appears to support such reforms.

Inadequate civic education

One line of criticism holds that citizens lack the basic education and decision-making skills necessary to be active participants in the political process. Such scholars as Jefferson, DeTocqueville and Bentham have argued that effective democracy requires that citizens be trained *in* democracy (DeTocqueville 1945; Pateman 1970). Barber argues simply that 'Information is indispensable to responsible exercise of citizenship and to the development of political judgment. Without civic education, democratic choice is little more than the expression and aggregation of private prejudices' (Barber 1984: 278).

Barber echoes a common view among media scholars and political scientists that ignorance on the part of the American voter severely constrains their ability to develop consistent political positions, 'to understand and evaluate policy options, and hence, to participate meaningfully in democratic politics' (Yankelovich 1991). Importantly, Barber appears to equate information and education with 'good' political judgement. From this perspective, polls that consistently find that most people cannot name their Congressional representative, let alone state or local representatives, might be considered proof that citizens are unable to participate effectively in the political process.

Whilst information may be necessary to engage the public in policy decisions, many argue that it is not sufficient. Yankelovich, for example, argues that this emphasis on the role of information is elitist, in that the traditional definition of 'well-informed' is to have the knowledge base of the governing elite. From this standpoint, civic education would imply the mere conveyance of facts from experts to the citizenry at large. Yankelovich wryly comments: 'The logic is this; they, the experts, are well informed; the public is poorly informed. Give the public more information, and it will agree with them' (Yankelovich 1991: 16).

From this perspective, the civic education required for democratic decision making involves not only the dissemination of information but also the building of the values underlying democratic decisions. Bellah *et al.* (1985), for example, argue that effective democracy requires that the public reconstruct value choices in civic or collective, rather than individualistic, terms. Etzioni (1988), Pateman (1970) and Putnam (1993a) concur that democratic renewal requires not merely information, but a shift in values at the most fundamental level. Finally, Yankelovich believes that civic education must develop the public's ability to understand and confront the value trade-offs inherent within policy choices.

Citizen apathy and inaction

A second line of argument regarding the failure of democracy is that citizens have become so alienated from and frustrated with the political process that they have become apathetic. Declining voter turnout and lack of attendance at public meetings are routinely heralded by scholars, politicians and public administrators as evidence of citizen apathy (Landers 1988; Chen 1992; Smith 1996). At the local level, this has seemingly been manifested by a decline in the traditions of civic association documented by DeTocqueville (1945). For example, Putnam cites declining membership in civic and fraternal associations as evidence of a withdrawal from the public sphere (Putnam 1995). Similarly, Blakely and Snyder (1997) contend that people are retreating from civic life to the insularity of gated communities.

Social science literature has advanced numerous hypotheses to explain citizen apathy, a detailed review of which is beyond the scope of this chapter. Political economists, for example, argue that citizen non-action is actually the result of a rational calculus comparing the costs and benefits of participation. Given that any single individual's effort is unlikely to make a difference, that it is usually difficult to exclude non-participants from enjoying the benefits of political action, and that the costs of participation are high, most citizens will choose to 'free ride' on the political activities of others (Downs 1957; Olsen 1965; Ostrom 1990; Miller 1997).

Critical theorists have argued that citizen apathy stems from a shift in focus and power away from communities and towards the world of work. Barber contends that this shift leads to apathy. As he argues, people are 'apathetic because they are powerless, not powerless because they are apathetic' (Barber 1984: 272). Similarly, Habermas (1979, 1989) argues that overcoming the oppression and enslavement of capitalism requires revitalising the public sphere through discourse.

The policy prescriptions for reducing citizen apathy range from technical interventions aiming to lower costs of participation, to more fundamental efforts to build political community. For example, the 'motor voter' law passed by Congress in 1993 attempted to lower the costs of voter registration by allowing people to register to vote at the same time as they conducted business at the state Department of Motor Vehicles. Public information and education campaigns, such as MTV's 'Rock the Vote' effort, encourage different sectors of the population to vote. Government efforts to encourage or require some sort of citizen participation in decision making at public meetings, although clearly cyclical (Creighton 1995), can be seen as another attempt to find a technical fix addressing citizen apathy.

On a deeper level, a number of scholars contend that to address political apathy, one must build effective local political communities based on neighbourhood organisations to bring about democratic renewal. For example, Barber argues that there is a need to reinvigorate our 'thin' (liberal/pluralist) democracy with a 'strong' democracy that combines democratic participation with meaningful association of citizens within a civic community:

> Community without participation first breeds unreflected consensus and conformity ... and finally engenders unitary collectivism of the kind that stifles citizenship and the autonomy on which political activity depends. Participation without community breeds mindless enterprise and undirected, competitive interest-mongering.
>
> (Barber 1984: 155)

Barber and others (Pateman 1970; Etzioni 1988; Ostrom 1990) believe that to embed democratic participation within the community requires that interest group politics be replaced with the politics of association within and among civic groups, at the neighbourhood level. The importance of networks of associations in a strong democracy is not a new idea. It was recognised as early as De Tocqueville's *Democracy in America:*

> The free institutions (associations/networks) which the inhabitants of the United States possess ... remind every citizen, and in a thousand ways that he lives in a society. They every instant impress upon his mind the notion that it is the duty as well as interest of men to make themselves useful to their fellow creatures.
>
> (De Tocqueville 1945: 112)

Much of the recent work on social capital highlights the importance of building strong civic associations as a means to reduce apathy and improve the democratic process (Coleman 1988; Putnam 1994 and Newton 1996). According to this literature, democratic processes function better when individuals operate within social networks of overlapping groups that have repeated interaction over time. Such networks of civic engagement increase confidence in social relations by increasing the costs of defection, foster norms of reciprocity, and improve information about the trustworthiness of individuals (Granovetter 1982; Ostrom 1990; Putnam 1993a). These values in turn facilitate the negotiation and compromise that democratic governance entails.

Need to connect government with the governed

The third line of criticism is that democracy is not functioning properly because there is a fundamental disconnection between citizens and their government. As Yankelovich describes: 'When the proper balance exists between the public and the nation's elite, our democracy works beautifully. When the balance is badly skewed, as in the present era, the system malfunctions, (Yankelovich 1991: 8).

Some have attributed this disconnection to the increased size and power of the bureaucracy (Niskanen 1971), or to the so-called 'iron triangle' of interest groups, administrative agents and legislators (Nordilinger 1983; Berry 1989; Stevens 1993). Others have argued that meaningful citizen involvement is barred by the information asymmetry between the governing elite and the general public (Campbell *et al.* 1960). Still others (Olsen 1965; Stigler 1971; Becker 1983; Mitchell and Munger 1991) contend that high communication and organisation costs bias the policy process to be more responsive to small, well-organised interests than to large, poorly organised groups.

Smith (1996) argues that much of the blame for this disconnection arises out of a perception of the buying and selling of political candidates. As Dionne states:

> Our system has become one long running advertisement against self-government. For many years we have been running down the public sector and public life. Voters doubt that elections give them any real control over what the government does, and half of them don't bother to cast ballots.
>
> (Dionne 1991: 1–2)

Many of the proposals for reuniting government with the governed call for a transfer of power from representatives and the business elite to 'ordinary' citizens. For example, campaign finance reform proposals attempt to restrict the influence of moneyed interest groups in the political process, and thus to give citizens a more central place in democratic processes. The initiative and referenda processes represent another attempt to give more direct power to citizens relative to the governing elite (Barber 1984). Efforts to 'devolve' decision making from the federal to the local level also aim to move government policy making closer to the individuals affected by policy decisions.

Many of these 'fixes' are little more than incremental and often politically symbolic attempts by politicians to engender public confidence in their ability to affect change. They seek to reduce the costs of citizen involvement in politics or the degree to which the complex language of government prevents citizens from engaging in political dialogue. The assumption is that reducing financial or information barriers will inevitably improve the level and quality of citizen government communication and interaction.

Many scholars (Pateman 1970; Bellah *et al.* 1985; Yankelovich 1991; Putnam 1993a; Fox and Miller 1995 and Bimber 1996), however, contend that a functioning democracy requires more than the removal of barriers to communication. It is not enough simply to provide citizens with the opportunity to become active in civic affairs: arcane public hearings held at midday are of little use to those who work. More fundamentally, political communication processes typically stand outside the daily consciousness of most citizens. Fox and Miller characterise the existing political process as the: 'Politics of hyperreality – a rapid sequence of images and symbols with unknown or uncertain referents racing through the public consciousness ... (where) simulation and media spectacle replace political debate' (Fox and Miller 1995: 43).

Building on Habermas (1975), Fox and Miller (1995) contend that the politics of hyperreality must be replaced by 'authentic discourse', which they characterise as sincere and honest, contextually or situationally based and conducted by willing, as opposed to coerced, participants with the goal of making a substantive contribution to the public good. Yankelovich echoes the call for a deeper discourse:

> For democracy to flourish, it is not enough to get out the vote.
> We need better public judgment, and we need to know how to

cultivate it. The public is not magically endowed with good judgment. Good judgment is something that must be worked at all the time and with great skill and effort. It does not exist automatically; it must be created.

(Yankelovich 1991: 11)

As with civic education, improvement in democracy is not simply a function of improving the mechanisms of communication, rather it requires developing a process that is *deliberative* in nature. Inherent in 'good' public judgement for Yankelovich and the authentic discourse of Fox and Miller is a focus on the value consequences of various policy options. Fixing democracy requires moving beyond mass opinion and snap judgements to thoughtful consideration of the important value conflicts inherent in political discourse.

Consequently, improving the connection between citizens and their representatives requires public debate to be *recursive*, with repeated dialogue regarding goals, and the value consequences of various options for achieving them. This type of repeated interaction between citizens and the governing elite will arguably provide opportunities for the process of 'working through' described by Yankelovich, wherein individuals acknowledge the value trade-offs inherent in political choices. It is not enough for citizens and government to have the opportunity simply to talk past one another. Democratic renewal requires what Barber terms 'dialogical' communication: cross-communication between citizens and citizens, and between citizens and public officials.

In sum, the literature on democratic participation suggests three broad areas of concern:

1 lack of education and civic value among the citizenry;
2 an apathetic public; and
3 a disconnection between the governing elite and the general public.

For each of these areas, we have identified a continuum of policy recommendations, which range from incremental modifications to our existing pluralist system, to more visionary recommendations for building a 'strong democracy'. This framework is summarised in Table 7.1. We now turn to the role that communications technology may play in improving democratic participation.

Table 7.1 Dimensions of democratic participation and potential responses

Impediments to democractic participation	Incremental modifications to pluralist system 'democracy'	Democratic renewal: building 'strong democracy'
Inadequate civic education	• Provide individuals with basic information about government and current events	• Help public 'come to judgement' through structured public debate of value choices
Apathetic citizenry	• Educate and encourage participation in political process • Facilitate interest group formation • Reduce costs of citizen interaction	• Facilitate formation of social and political community groups • Build levels of trust and generalised norms of reciprocity between citizens
Disconnection between citizens and their government	• Encourage citizen 'voice' to improve official understanding of range of preferences • Decentralise or localise policy making • Reduce costs of participation • Level the playing field between elite and less advantaged individuals or groups	• Foster 'deliberative' communication between citizens and government • Facilitate recursive and dialogical patterns of interaction

Telecommunications technologies and democratic renewal

The internet has been argued to increase the opportunity for citizens and the governing elite to communicate more effectively, and at lower cost. Whilst these capabilities clearly facilitate the types of incremental democratic reforms we have identified, it is less clear whether the internet will foster the development of more thoughtful, civic-minded and deliberative patterns of communication.

The internet and civic education

The internet would seem to be a capable tool for providing citizens with civic and political information. For example, new telecommunications technologies can provide citizens with more information in more easily accessible formats than traditional formats. Many projects are designed to reacquaint citizens with basic information about how government works and how individuals can influence the process. (See, for example, the California Voter Foundation web site, www.calvote.org.) The technology is also capable of disseminating political positions and campaign-related information to voters. Several candidates, political parties and non-partisan groups have already begun to exploit these possibilities.

To the extent that democratic renewal requires citizens to focus on the fundamental value choices in a democracy, however, civic education efforts that merely acquaint the public with the procedural rules of the democracy are insufficient. Instead, civic education must inculcate individuals with the ideals of a commonwealth, a sense of the common good and civic responsibility, by promoting activities that require confrontation with difficult value choices and the consequences of those choices. It is possible that the internet can assist in this process, given its capability for two-way, mediated and recursive communication which could aid confrontation of such difficult value choices. Such deliberative and recursive communication between citizens and government, however, is a different proposition from simply providing information about civic affairs or current policy proposals.

Building 'virtual' community

The most important step in overcoming apathy is the development of effective political community at the local level. It is possible that the internet may foster the development of political community by increasing citizen-to-citizen communication. Clearly, the internet may facilitate lower-cost communication through chat rooms and list-serve technologies. The crucial question, however, is whether use of these technologies fosters stable 'cybercommunites' that bring people together in sustained civic relationships, as opposed to encouraging fleeting or anonymous social contacts.

On a more fundamental level, the issue is whether the internet can effectively develop social capital, and particularly the trust and norms of generalised reciprocity that many believe are the essential components of effective community. It is not clear whether the internet is an appropriate tool for this task. For example, evidence from simulated public good experiments suggests that computer-mediated communication may decrease levels of trust or reciprocity when compared to face-to-face interaction (Palfrey and Rosenthal 1988; Sell and Wilson 1991 and 1992; Rocco and Warglien 1995). In addition, Berry *et al.* (1993), in their study of urban participation, argue that *face-to-face* communication is necessary for citizen participation to be effective. In a meta-analysis of experiments from 1959 to 1992, Sally (1995) found that face-to-face communication significantly raised the co-operation rate, on average by more than 45 per cent (Ostrom 1998).

Bringing citizens close to government

The internet may be a way to reduce the distance between the governing elite and the citizenry. A key barrier to the revitalisation of democracy is that the 'experts' and 'special interests' simply have more information than the general public. It is certainly possible that this new communication medium will level the informational playing field for the average citizen. The ease of e-mail also potentially opens up access to decision makers. It seems logical, therefore, that the internet could reduce the cost of communication between citizens and government.

The more fundamental issue, of course, is whether the internet can foster the *deliberative* type of communication between citizens and government that Yankelovich (1991), Bellah *et al.* (1985) and Fox and Miller (1995) believe is necessary for true democratic renewal. Here the evidence is less encouraging. For example, Guthrie *et al.* (1990) found that public discourse over the Public Electronic Network in Santa Monica, California, came to be dominated by a small and vocal group of citizens in a very short period of time, with elected officials largely absent from the discussions. This suggests that deliberative communication by electronic means may be difficult to sustain. Barber makes this point clear in his discussion of electronic balloting. As he argues for such a system, he also warns that:

> The objective is not to canvass opinion or to take a straw poll, but to catalyze discussion and to nurture empathetic forms of reasoning. Soliciting instant votes on every conceivable issue from an otherwise uniformed audience that has neither deliberated nor debated an issue would be the death of democracy.
>
> (Barber 1984: 289–90)

In sum, the internet, at least in theory, creates the *opportunity* to improve communications and reconnect citizens with their representatives, other citizens and democracy. It does offer genuinely orig-inal possibilities, including greater levels of interaction, easier access to information, and support for group-based communication. Whether and how governmental applications of these technological capabilities will affect democratic processes will nonetheless depend on how they are designed and used – the social shaping of the tech-nology. To that end, we turn to some empirical data on the extent to which existing implementations of world wide web sites accord with the demands for democratic renewal.

Evidence from California municipal web pages

To examine the extent to which advanced communications tech-nologies enhance the features of democratic participation outlined above, we turn to evidence from California municipal web pages. By examining actual uses of the internet, this analysis fills a gap in the literature concerning democratic renewal. This inattention to existing applications may be due, at least in part, to an excessive focus on the internet's capability of providing information and facil-itating horizontal and vertical communication at greatly reduced cost. On this level, the internet so obviously furthers what we have termed *incremental* modifications that its value is simply taken for granted. Our evidence suggests, however, that the current shaping of the technology is unlikely to support meaningful and widespread changes to local democratic processes.

Methodology

The focus of our research is on a particular portion of the internet, namely municipal world wide web sites, which we define as any site, either publicly or privately provided, that includes information concerning a specific locality (Weare *et al.* 1999). We have chosen to focus on cities because they are governments with which citizens inter-act most intimately as recipients of basic governmental services (e.g. road repair, policing) and as direct participants in the democratic process. In autumn 1996, an extensive search identified 135 sites covering 118 of California's 460 cities (Hale 1997). A subsequent investigation in the summer of 1997 found that the number of cities with web site addresses had increased 91% to 214 (Weare *et al.* 1999). By 1997, a total of 290 web site addresses were identified. Sixty-one cities had two or more sites, and eleven had three or more different sites describing some aspect of the locality.[1]

We found a tremendous variation in the information available on the web sites. The cities of Santa Monica (pen.ci.santa-monica.ca.us), San Jose (www.ipac.net/csj/), Palo Alto (www.city.palo-alto.ca.us) and West Hollywood (www.ci.west-hollywood.ca.us), for example, provide the user with rich information on virtually every type of city and civic function imaginable, and allow users to ask questions of city staff electronically on a wide range of issues. In contrast, many sites are so small and elementary that they are in reality nothing more than a type-written page electronically presented. For example, Carlsbad (www.carslbad.ca.us) and Yorba Linda (www. yorbalinda.org) provide users with only basic city information, such as a city description. The majority of sites range between these two extremes, providing the most basic city information but without extensive mechanisms and detail required for visitors to conduct basic business on the web.

The rapid spread of this technology, in combination with the variation in quality, suggests that we are confronted with the problem of examining a moving target. What is interesting, however, is the consistency of a city web page once it is designed. Of the web pages in existence in 1996, only a small number appeared substantially different by 1997. Whilst information within the web page was generally kept current, the type of information presented and the design of the web page changed little over the period of a year. For example, cities generally present current minutes of city council meetings on the web page, but few cities expanded on the level of detail presented within the minutes.

Results

The first requisite for democratic renewal we identified is improved civic education. From a standpoint of incremental improvements, the goal is to provide citizens with more information about basic civic functions. Doing so will, presumably, provide citizens with the tools necessary to become effective in the political process. Web pages can provide a wide range of different types of specific government information. This information can be seen as an attempt to inform citizens of the day-to-day workings of government. Providing this information to citizens and, more importantly, local interest or community groups, presumably also lowers information, monitoring and transaction costs between groups. This information then serves both a civic education and a horizontal communication function.

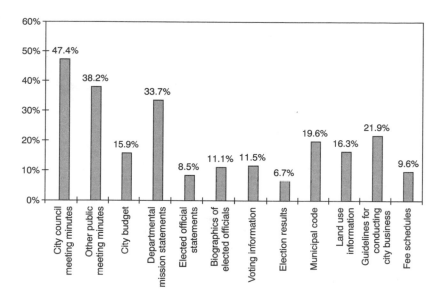

Figure 7.1 Percentage of sites providing information on governmental operations

Source: The authors.

Figure 7.1 shows discouraging results regarding the provision of city government information. For example, fewer than one-half of all sites provided information on city council or other public meeting minutes, and fewer than one-fifth provided information regarding the city budget. There was very little information regarding elected officials, voting, election results or fee schedules. Thus, municipal web pages do not appear to provide even basic civic information, a role for which they would appear to be ideally suited. As such, a citizen or interest group attempting to learn more about civic affairs might not be able to rely on a municipal web page for basic civic education.

The second avenue towards democratic renewal is to strengthen civic associations and build social capital by facilitating horizontal communication and interaction between groups. From a standpoint of incrementalist change, web pages might lower information, monitoring and transaction costs between citizen groups. In the content analysis, coders were asked to gather information on six different types of local organisations. These include grass-roots advocacy groups (e.g. Greenpeace, Sierra Club), neighbourhood-oriented organisations (e.g. Neighbourhood Watch, block clubs), city-sponsored citizen organisations (e.g. leadership councils, civic pride groups), fraternal/social organisations (e.g. Elks Club), charities (e.g. Salvation Army) and finally religious congregations. It is possible on the web page to provide the following levels of information about each type of organisation:

1   none;
2   information only;
3   links to the civic group's web page or an e-mail address; and
4   both information and links or e-mail.

The results presented in Figure 7.2 are not encouraging. At most, 30 per cent of city web pages contained any information about these organisations. Only in the case of religious congregations were both links and information apparent in more than 10 per cent of the cities. Only 3 per cent of sites provided information and links to grass-roots organisations, and only 8 per cent did so about neighbourhood, fraternal and social organisations.

Beyond providing links to community organisations, achieving more fundamental democratic renewal requires building a rich network of associations and social networks to develop the norms of reciprocity and trust. As seen in Figure 7.3, however, very few city web pages provided such a rich network of horizontal communication channels. Only 4.4 per cent of all sites provided more than

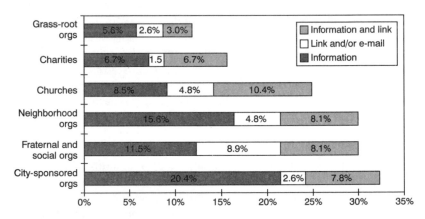

Figure 7.2 Information and links to local groups
Source: The authors.

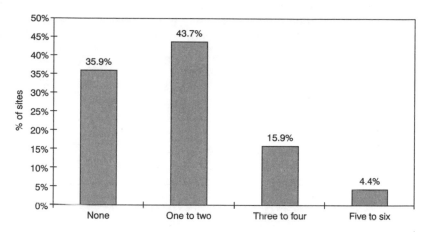

Figure 7.3 Number of horizontal communication links supported
Source: The authors.

four horizontal communication channels. More than one-third of all cities provided no horizontal communication links whatsoever, and 44 per cent provided only one or two links.

Alternatively, horizontal communications could be supported electronically through the use of 'chat room' functions or with electronic bulletin boards. As Barber contends, 'democracy must have its local talk shop' (1984: 268). Table 7.2 shows that municipal web sites are particularly thin from a standpoint of horizontal communications: only 2.6 per cent provide chat rooms, and only 9.3 per cent have electronic bulletin boards. These results suggest that municipal sites, as designed currently, are unlikely to foster social capital.

The third factor we examine is vertical communication between citizens and government. At the most basic level, the argument is that the provision of information about government offices will lead to a closer relationship or connection between the two sides. Web sites were coded as to whether they provided information about nine different types of local government offices, and for the appearance of information on county, state, federal offices and special districts. The results are presented in Figure 7.4.

The results in this area are somewhat encouraging. More than 50 per cent of all sites contained some information regarding the major city functional departments. It should be noted that the single most common area of information provision was cultural and leisure

Table 7.2 Percentage of sites with two-way
communication capabilities

Type of communication	%
Horizontal communications	
Chat rooms	2.6
Electronic bulletin boards	9.3
Vertical communications	
Comment boxes	16.3
Electronic forms	20.7

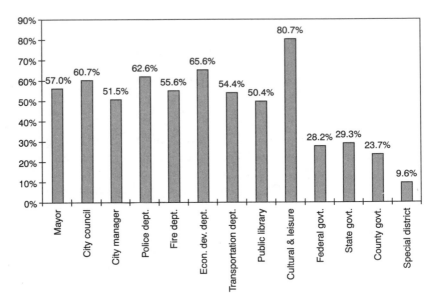

Figure 7.4 Percentage of sites providing information on government
offices

Source: The authors.

information, provided by 80.7 per cent of all sites. Many fewer sites
provided information about other levels of government, such as federal, state or county governments, and less than 10 per cent of all sites
provided information about special districts. As seen in Figure 7.5,
over 40 per cent of the sites provided a rich array of information, covering eight or more of the thirteen offices surveyed. Nevertheless, the
results are quite uneven with a large percentage of sites, over 35 per
cent, providing either no information or covering less than four offices.

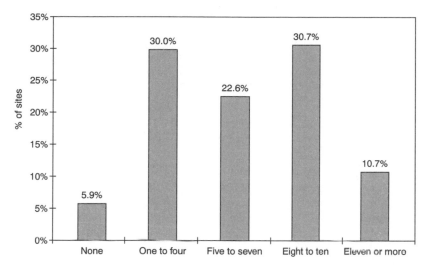

Figure 7.5 Number of vertical communication links supported
Source: The authors.

From a more fundamental standpoint, it has been argued that to narrow the gap between citizen and the governing elite requires deliberative (both recursive and dialogical) communication. At the very minimum, deliberative communication would seem to require that citizens can contact their elected or government officials directly, through phone or mail contact information (a directory function). Better would be the presence of e-mail channels to elected officials and city staff, through the presence of general comment boxes or through electronic forms.

This does not mean that the presence of e-mail, comment boxes or electronic forms *guarantees* deliberative communication. It is quite possible that no deliberative-type communication will occur, even if citizens have the ability to contact officials through electronic means. Whilst this question invites further study, it is enough, for our purposes, to say that without some ability to contact city officials electronically, the internet cannot foster deliberative communication.

Table 7.3 suggests that city web pages generally are not using electronic communication capabilities to their fullest potential for facilitating deliberative communication. A substantial number of sites did not provide communications access to the mayor (44.1 per cent), the city council (40.7 per cent) or to the city manager (49.6 per cent).

Table 7.3 Percentage of sites offering communication access to city officials

	Mayor (%)	City council (%)	City manager (%)
No communications access	44.1	40.7	49.6
Traditional 'phone book' access			
Mail address	37.8	37.8	33.3
Contact names			
At least one	51.5	52.6	39.3
Two or more	3.3	18.1	7.4
Telephone numbers			
At least one	44.1	48.5	45.6
Two or more	5.9	9.3	2.6
Electronic access			
E-mail			
At least one	17.8	21.1	13.7
Two or more	0.7	4.1	2.2
Links	13.3	14.1	11.9

Those sites that did attempt to facilitate communication concentrated predominately on traditional 'phone book' functions, providing a mail address or a single contact name or telephone number. Few, however, provided more than a single contact name or telephone number, and less than one-fifth provided e-mail or links to public officials.[2] In addition, as summarised in Table 8.2 above, municipal web sites do not support alternative avenues for vertical communication. Only 16.3 per cent have comment boxes, and 20.7 per cent have electronic forms that can be submitted directly to city agencies.

Conclusions

The results of this study are not encouraging. We have identified three impediments to democratic participation: lack of civic education, citizen apathy, and the disconnection between citizens and their representatives. Democratic theorists and political reformers have suggested a number of reforms to address these ills. Some reforms call for incremental changes to pluralistic democracy, whilst others call for a more fundamental development of participative democratic processes. We argue that internet technologies clearly have the potential to foster incremental changes to existing pluralistic institutions. In contrast, we contend that it is far less certain that the internet will nurture the rich network of social relations and discourse required to develop Barber's vision of a strong democracy.

We did find several exemplar sites that creatively explore the full potential of the internet to further municipal governance.[3] They facilitate access to information of interest to local citizens and provide communication channels between citizens and their representatives and among citizens. The very best also provide information and access to community groups and incorporate chat rooms and other technologies that may enrich local political discourse.

Unfortunately, such sites appear rare. The evidence from California indicates that an important feature of the internet is rarely used in ways that can reasonably be thought to lead to incremental reform, let alone democratic renewal. In general, information provision is patchy and the level of interactivity supported does not improve significantly on the telephone. Moreover, when we examined more fundamental uses of technology that foster political community through deliberative and value-infused communication, we found that the current city use of web technology does little, if anything, to foster this type of democratic revitalisation.

Future research is needed to explore the factors that led to the development of these exemplar sites, to understand the extent to which citizens are actually using the technology, and the effects of the technology on the quality of political debate. These results may also serve as a baseline for comparing new developments in the social shaping of technology over time.

Notes

1 The data presented below are from the 290 sites identified in the summer of 1997. Three trained coders conducted a structured content analysis on the 290 identified sites, coding 106 variables having to do with the types of information provided, the level of interactivity, and the general design and emphasis of each site. Twenty sites were not found by the coders and were eliminated from the date set. Inter-coder reliability was acceptable. Using Krippendorf's (1980) alpha, questions scored on a nominal scale had an alpha of .69, and questions scored on an ordinal scale had an alpha of .76. These scores indicate that the observed level of agreement was 69 per cent and 76 per cent, respectively, above that which would be achieved by pure chance.

2 Although these results cover only three government offices, the patterns of communication for other city departments were similar.

3 See Musso *et al.* 1998 for further discussion of exemplar sites.

8 Closed Circuit Television and Information Age policy processes

C. William R. Webster

Introduction

Of central importance to a book entitled 'Digital Democracy' are the complex relationships between new Information and Communication Technologies (ICTs) and democratic structures and procedures. Often discussions about democracy in the Information Age focus on the potential offered by internet-based applications for improved democratic practices, and in particular, improved citizen 'input' into the democratic process. Unlike these discussions and many of the chapters in this book, this chapter is not concerned directly with the impact of internet-related ICTs on democratic processes. Rather, it offers an analysis of the policy processes surrounding the widespread diffusion of Closed Circuit Television (CCTV) surveillance cameras in public places across the UK. Thus, whilst the other chapters are mainly concerned with improvements in democratic 'inputs' resulting from the diffusion of new technology, the focus of this chapter is a new technological 'output' of the current political, policy and democratic processes. At the centre of this chapter is an ICT-intensive policy 'tool' used to meet policy objectives and service requirements, rather than a technological tool designed directly to improve democratic procedures. CCTV is a tool used primarily to detect and deter crime and reduce the Fear of Crime (FOC); nevertheless, as a policy tool provided by the democratic agencies of the state, CCTV highlights the interrelationships between new technology and policy processes. These processes include the role and importance of political rhetoric and public discourse and are of central importance to contemporary democratic practice. The term 'digital' or 'electronic' democracy in this chapter is relevant in its broadest sense and goes beyond the narrow concerns of direct citizen participation to incorporate the wider importance of political discourse, policy making and service delivery in democratic processes.

The widespread introduction of CCTV across UK public space is occurring in response to actual and perceived rises in levels of crime and the FOC, and the apparent ability of surveillance cameras to help prevent and deter criminal activity. Their introduction is the result of both a demand by citizens for the right to personal and communal safety, and a desire by politicians and democratic bodies to demonstrate that they are actively tackling the problems of crime, disorder and other anti-social behaviour. CCTV therefore represents the introduction of a highly symbolic, technologically based tool in the 'fight against crime' and a public policy process in which satisfying citizens' expectations and demands is central to the legitimation of policy and the distribution of services. What is absent from these policy processes, however, is any significant public debate about the need for, and the implications of, installing sophisticated surveillance systems so widely in society. Limitations in the nature of public discourse suggest that the policy process has been manipulated to reassert the democratic legitimacy of the existing institutions of democratic governance. The provision of CCTV, it is therefore argued, provides evidence of democratic institutions exploiting the application of new technology to help renew their legitimacy and thereby re-establish their place at the centre of the democratic polity.

The objective of this chapter is to use CCTV as a case study to discuss the nature and evolution of policy and democratic processes in the Information Age. The key aims of the chapter are: to highlight the rapid uptake of CCTV in 'public' places; to identify issues arising from this uptake; to discuss government policy and policy process surrounding the provision of CCTV; and to discuss the changing relations in society arising from the widespread use of sophisticated surveillance technology. In particular, the chapter will discuss changing relations between citizens and the state, and the importance and role of political rhetoric and public discourse in providing new technology in democratic settings.

The uptake of CCTV

Since the mid-1990s, the UK has been in the throes of an unprecedented 'surveillance revolution', where CCTV has rapidly been installed in various 'public' locations (Webster 1996). One group of researchers even argues that 'Britain now has more wide area CCTV systems geared towards surveying the public behaviour of citizens in public places than any other advanced capitalist nation' (Graham *et al.* 1996: 1).

A typical CCTV system will consist of a series of strategically located cameras, networked by a dedicated 'closed circuit' telecommunications infrastructure to a control room, where trained operatives view events live on banks of monitors. The police can be informed of incidents as they happen, and video images can be recorded to be used later by police to aid investigation and as evidence in the prosecution of suspects. Modern surveillance systems convey near television quality images, are operative at night and can focus on the smallest of detail.

The CCTV systems discussed in this chapter are those unique 'public' systems that survey public locations (locations to which citizens have free and unhindered access) and are financed by institutions in the public sector, in particular the democratic institutions of governance. A number of commentators have noted the widespread diffusion of CCTV systems in town and city centres across the UK (see, for example, Fyfe and Bannister 1996; Graham 1996; Graham et al. 1996). Although initially the majority of large-scale public systems were located in town and city centres, diffusion has now moved beyond metropolitan areas into a wide variety of public locations (Webster 1996). CCTV systems can now be found in schools, hospitals, libraries, car parks, along motorways and in residential and rural areas. Home and Scottish Office statistics (Table 8.1 and Figure 8.1) show that the government's 'CCTV Challenge Competition' has contributed £50 million to nearly 700 new schemes across all regions of the UK. The Home Office estimates that the competitions have resulted in over 10,000 new cameras being installed in public locations (Home Office 1995b). This is in addition to the many public systems funded independently of the Home Office, and numerous 'private' surveillance systems installed in a wide variety of locations, including banks, shops, offices, petrol stations, shopping centres and business parks.

The speed with which sophisticated CCTV surveillance systems have been installed in public places across the UK is unprecedented, and without doubt a feature of the 1990s. Part of the explanation for this 'camera-mania' is the belief that the cameras meet their stated goal to 'help prevent and detect crime . . . (and) . . . also deter criminals and reassure the public' (Home Office 1994: 3). This has enabled CCTV to be promoted and marketed to the general public as an effective technological tool to combat crime. In Glasgow, for example, as Figure 8.2 illustrates, crime has fallen dramatically since the introduction of CCTV. Statistical evidence such as this shows that installing CCTV results in reductions in recorded crime and

Table 8.1 Summary of successful bids in CCTV Challenge Competition

	Round 1 1995–6	Round 2 1996–7	Round 3 1997–8	Round 4 1998–9	Total
Number of successful bids	111	291	218	55	675
Amount awarded (£000)	n/a	18,989	16,860	3,092	38,941
Total capital cost of schemes (£000)	n/a	45,016	40,753	6,200*	92,000*

Note: *indicates estimation

Sources: Adapted from Home Office 1995a and 1996b, 1997, 1998; Scottish Office 1996a, 1997 and 1998

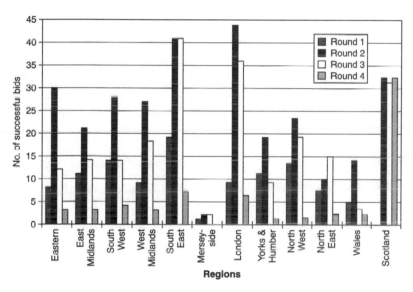

Figure 8.1 Successful bids in the CCTV Challenge Competition: number of schemes by region

Sources: adapted from Home Office 1995a, 1996b, 1997 and 1998, and Scottish Office 1996a, 1997 and 1998

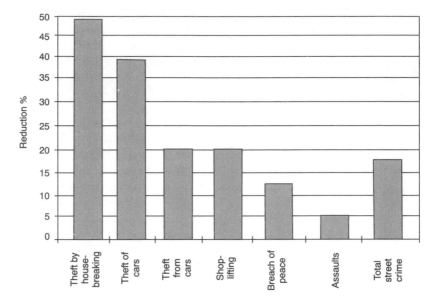

Figure 8.2 Crime reduction and Glasgow CityWatch (14 months to end of February 1996)

Source: adapted from Strathclyde Police 1996

reinforces the belief and perception that CCTV works as a tool for achieving crime reduction.

Government policy, political rhetoric and public discourse

The new Labour government has continued the previous Conservative administration's support for CCTV through financial assistance, policy guidance and political rhetoric. The Crime Prevention Agency Unit of the Home Office and the Crime Prevention Unit of the Scottish Office are funding CCTV systems through the aforementioned 'CCTV Challenge Competition'. The competitions are run annually (a summary of awards to date are illustrated in Table 8.1 and Figure 8.1) and make contributions to the capital costs of schemes where it can be demonstrated that there is a need for CCTV, where 'community partners' including the police, local authorities and local businesses are involved in provision, and where the majority of capital costs are paid by private sources. The competition requires that bids for funding demonstrate how future running costs will be met, that a code of practice concerning the use of cameras exists and that appropriate evaluation procedures are in place.

Financial assistance has been backed up through policy and operational guidance. The Home Office and Scottish Office have both published detailed guidance documents (Home Office 1994; Scottish Office 1996b) giving advice on the siting, design and operation of CCTV systems. These documents are designed to give those considering installing CCTV a basic knowledge of the subject, its advantages and pitfalls, and a plan of how best to proceed in installing the most suitable system. Regulation of CCTV schemes has been kept to a minimum: there is no licensing system concerning the location of installation, and there is no binding legislation regulating who may use them, or how they may be used. Whilst codes of practice (see, for example, LGIU 1996) may be a requirement for securing Home Office funding, they are voluntary. There is no legal requirement to draw up a code, no agreed formula advising on the content of the code, and no way of ensuring that it is being implemented. Consequently, the codes vary considerably in size and content (Bulos and Sarno 1996). At present, it could be said that the CCTV policy arena is practically unregulated, and at best only voluntary self-regulation exists.

Operating guidance and financial assistance has been reinforced with political rhetoric. Scottish Office Home Affairs Minister Henry McLeish, when announcing the results of the 1998–9 Scottish Office Challenge Competition, said 'we are giving CCTV our strongest support because there can be no doubt that CCTV works ... (and) ... most crucially for me, CCTV helps reduce the fear of crime on the streets' (McLeish 1998: 11). The view that CCTV is a successful tool for crime prevention and deterrence has been widely disseminated across society, and accordingly there is widespread support for CCTV amongst politicians, policy makers and the general public. Amongst the general public there is a perception that crime and the FOC is rising. Findings from the 1996 British Crime Survey (Home Office 1996a) show that three quarters of those surveyed (mistakenly) believed that recorded crime is rising and felt that they were more likely to be a victim of crime. Public perception surveys such as those conducted by the Home Office (Honess and Charman 1992) and prospective operators show clearly that the general public perceive CCTV as a highly effective tool in reducing crime and the FOC. For example, research carried out in the Easterhouse district of Glasgow shows that 95 per cent of local residents were 'satisfied' or 'very satisfied' with the introduction of a CCTV system, and 70

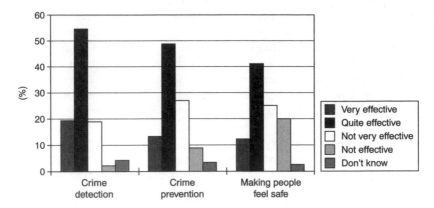

Figure 8.3 Public perception of the effectiveness of CCTV

Source: adapted from Honess and Charman 1992: 19

per cent felt that the introduction of a CCTV system would 'improve' or 'greatly improve' the quality of life in their area (Ross and Hood 1998). Similarly, research conducted by the Home Office in 1992 and illustrated in Figure 8.3 shows that over 60 per cent of the general public surveyed perceived CCTV to be 'very' or 'quite' effective. This research also found that only 6 per cent of those surveyed were worried about the presence of surveillance cameras.

There are two distinct features of the public discourse surrounding the provision of CCTV in the UK. Firstly, that the overwhelming public support is unquestionable, and secondly, that public debate about the introduction of CCTV in public places is limited. To date, the political rhetoric on CCTV has focused on the effectiveness of CCTV technology in addressing the rising levels of crime and the FOC, and this is the view that has been disseminated across society. CCTV is not criticised, as only 'citizens with something to hide have something to fear'. This dominant view has stifled public discourse and curtailed debate on the use and implications of CCTV. The belief that society needs these systems has overridden dissenters who question their impacts and effectiveness. The narrowness of current discourse suggests that debate has been dominated by political rhetoric and perhaps shaped by those with a vested interest in promoting the technology, including the police, central and local government, retailers and equipment manufacturers.

It is thus apparent that political communication, in the form of policy statements, political discourse and advertising, has shaped the CCTV policy agenda into a situation amenable to CCTV provision, or, as Sir Geoffrey Vickers (1995) would have argued, that society's 'appreciative setting' has shifted position so that the widespread surveillance of citizens in public locations by the state is acceptable. More recently, there are signs that political discourse about the provision of CCTV is starting to broaden. Two recent reports, one for the European Parliament and the other by the House of Lords, question the role and effects of CCTV, showing that at the policy-making level at least debate is starting to widen. The Scientific and Technological Options Assessment (STOA) unit report for the European Parliament (STOA 1998) categorises CCTV as a 'technology of political control' used to enhance policing *and* internal control. The report warns against the 'immense power' of surveillance technology, pointing out that it can be used for both law enforcement and advanced state suppression. It therefore recommends that the European Union develop appropriate mechanisms for democratically accountable and transparent political control of new CCTV surveillance technology. The House of Lords Select Committee report on 'Digital Images' (House of Lords 1998) stresses the importance of public support for the continued diffusion of CCTV. This report argues that currently 'public acceptance is based on a limited, and partly inaccurate knowledge of the functions and capabilities of CCTV systems' (House of Lords 1998: 4.8) and is hence fragile and reversible. The report proposes tighter governmental control over CCTV in order to meet the requirement of continued public support. The Lords' concern is that limitations in the extent of public debate and understanding could undermine its diffusion. Thus they suggest that the government should play a greater part in leading public debate: 'we want to see public acceptance of surveillance ... this is more likely to be the case if there is a wider public debate on the issues involved, and we consider that the government should provide such a debate' (House of Lords 1998: 4.22). What this report highlights is that through the shaping and leading of political discourse, the government will be able to set the policy agendas surrounding CCTV and thereby manage diffusion. The sophisticated use of political communication to shape and lead discourse implies that policy making is a top down process in which policy and discourse are determined by policy specialists and political elites. Habermas (1989) would argue that the domination of political discourse by government is resulting in the erosion of the traditional public 'sphere' where citizens were able to discuss political ideas and formulate their political identity. In this perspective, the lack of public space to engage in political discourse will ultimately lead to democratic crisis.

CCTV: some issues

The diffusion of CCTV is not just about reducing crime and the FOC, it also plays an important role in ensuring societal order and deterring anti-social behaviour. Just as criminal actions are deterred, so too are general misdemeanours such as littering and loitering. Beyond its primary purpose, CCTV is regarded as a cost-effective way of dealing with a range of problems, including vandalism, drunkenness, harassment, prostitution, loitering, driving offences and disorderly behaviour. CCTV also provides police forces with greater flexibility in the management of their resources. It enables the police to respond to incidents more quickly and redistribute their manpower more effectively. CCTV has also been credited with revitalising the financial health of town centres by encouraging shoppers and tourists to use local amenities (Graham *et al.* 1996). The provision of CCTV is therefore not solely about reducing crime. It is part of a wider debate on law and order policy, encompassing the provision of policing and law and order services.

Whilst CCTV has proved to be very popular, its introduction raises important issues for contemporary democratic practice. These issues derive from questions raised about the ability of the cameras actually to reduce crime, and the unknown impacts that they have on individual behaviour. The effectiveness of CCTV in reducing crime – the premise on which it has been provided – should not be taken as fact. Doubts have been raised about whether CCTV can reduce crime and, if it does, on the effects upon neighbouring localities as displacement occurs (Short and Ditton 1995; House of Lords 1998). Short and Ditton also question the way in which statistics cited to demonstrate the effectiveness of CCTV are collected and the evaluation of systems is carried out. For them, the remarkable cuts in crime figures cited to back up the effectiveness of CCTV must be treated with considerable caution.

Those critical of CCTV argue that its introduction is irreversibly altering relations between individuals and the state. Such critics see CCTV primarily as a tool for maintaining social order in a technologically driven surveillance society (see, for example, Davies 1996; STOA 1998). In ensuring social order, CCTV impinges upon individual basic civil liberties, and in particular individual rights to personal privacy and the right to go about daily lawful business without hindrance by the state. The introduction of CCTV affects citizens' rights, and hence the citizen–state relationship, in a variety of ways (see Webster 1998 for a discussion about CCTV and citizens' rights). By preventing and deterring crime, CCTV enhances civil rights by reinforcing individuals' right to freedom of movement and security in surveyed areas. On the other hand, it can equally be argued that CCTV jeopardises rights. The degree to which the use of CCTV contributes to a loss of individual privacy and to unwarranted levels of individual surveillance is a concern recognised by civil liberties groups (SCCL 1994; National Council 1989). The personal freedom 'to go about one's legal business without intrusion from the state' is defined by Harry Street (1972) as *the* fundamental civil liberty. Within this liberty are the civil rights to privacy and the freedom of movement. Privacy is a broad concept that involves a whole range of human concerns about various forms of intrusive behaviour. The extension of state surveillance, monitoring and supervision capacity, through the use of new ICTs, highlights a general fear of the kind of continuous surveillance portrayed in George Orwell's classic *Nineteen Eighty-Four* (1965).

Alongside issues raised about privacy are concerns about the civil right to freedom of movement. CCTV systems give the surveyors considerable power to decide who has unhindered access to an area and who deserves surveillance. Decisions about who to observe derive from the operatives' perceptions about links between visual appearance and the behaviour of people. Instantaneous decisions about who to monitor may be made by association or appearance, rather than evidence. Consequently, individuals who find themselves continually under surveillance may choose not to enter those areas where surveillance occurs. The use of surveillance technology in this way could result in the social segregation of public places by discouraging unwanted or undesirable citizens' access and freedom of movement in public spaces (Davies 1990). Presumably these individuals would include those who might discourage shoppers and tourists, such as drunkards, vandals and loiterers.

The application of new technology for social surveillance and control is not a new perspective (see, for example, Gandy 1994; Lyon 1994; Davies 1996). Foucault's (1977) work around 'disciplinary surveillance' in society would suggest that CCTV is a general expression of power, a new technological tool of the disciplinary network designed to provide obedient citizens. Giddens' (1985) work also points to the application of new technology as reinforcing the administrative power of the state to regulate the activity of citizens. Clearly the application of CCTV has fundamental implications for the evolution of the citizen–state relationship. This is because CCTV is not just a policy tool for ensuring law and order but is also a tool controlling citizens and society. The new citizen–state relationship is characterised by the state surveillance of citizens and the acceptance of this as the norm. The extent of this surveillance has led some commentators to note that we are entering an era that could be called the 'surveillance society' (Davies 1996; Lyon 1994).

If we look more closely at the ability of CCTV to reduce crime, its effects on civil liberties, and its implications for human behaviour, then the question of why we are adopting CCTV surveillance technology so widely in society must be asked. Furthermore, this question raises additional important issues about the extent of rationality in the policy process, the unequivocal support for CCTV, and the limitations in the extent of public discourse on the use and impacts of its application (Webster 1996).

The future of CCTV: Bigger, Better Brother?

Rapid advances in surveillance technology over the last decade have meant that CCTV surveillance systems in public places are commonplace today. Although the uptake of these systems has been extremely quick, they are comparatively simple and are likely to be integrated with far more sophisticated technology in the not too distant future. Current systems are relatively 'dumb' in that they require operators, analysis of incidents, and because offenders remain anonymous. Developments in CCTV technology will introduce more 'intelligent' systems. In the future, CCTV surveillance systems are likely to become more computerised through the increased use of image databases and image-recognition software, and they are likely to be more integrated as separate systems are networked together.

One development that is already well advanced is the use of recognition software. Roadside surveillance cameras using basic image-recognition technology are currently being used in British ports and the city of London to scan and recognise all traffic. Sophisticated facial-recognition software, which can identify individuals and match them against details held on computer databases, are currently under development and are likely to be introduced in the next five to ten years. One system already being tested is Virtual Interactive Policing (VIP), which enables police officers to scan a crowd or street and automatically cross-match the figures against a database of known offenders (May 1996). To be fully effective, a national facial-recognition system would require access to a large database of digitised faces and personal records. Although such a database does not yet exist, Simon Davies, Director of Privacy International, argues that the Driver and Vehicle Licensing Agency's plans for a smart-card driving licence incorporating a digitised image of the driver's face could be utilised for this purpose (Davies 1996).

Advanced computerisation allowing facial and image recognition, and the extensive use of databases are likely to be allied to the widespread networking of disparate CCTV systems. A number of manufacturers already market remote surveillance packages that use the public telephone network to transmit images to a central control room. In the future, the integration of neighbouring CCTV systems is likely to take advantage of the economies of scale by using shared control rooms and personnel. The potential for a national recognition, monitoring and tracking system based around existing CCTV systems appears to be an achievable vision. The integration of disparate CCTV systems, coupled with advances in computerisation, could one day create intelligent systems much closer to Orwell's 'Big Brother' than the current systems. If this is the case, then the current uptake of CCTV is perhaps just the first stage in this scenario.

CCTV and policy processes in the Information Age

Because citizens desire reduced crime and improved safety, it can be argued that government, through the application of new ICTs, is delivering the services citizens want. It follows, therefore, that in responding to citizens' demands, politicians and government are able to reassert their right to represent the interests of citizens and repopularise themselves through the application of new technology. Although new CCTV surveillance technology is being used to reduce crime and improve general policing, the application of such technology provides opportunities to reinforce existing power structures in society, including current democratic structures and procedures. The perceived success of CCTV in reducing crime and its general popularity demonstrates that politicians and policy makers are acting responsively to public demand for greater safety. It also demonstrates that democratic institutions of governance can reassert their position as the focal point of contemporary democracy. This leads us to ask whether the traditional, constitutional, democratic model of the polity is reasserting itself through the application of new technology, or whether it is being reinvented in an amended form. (See Horrocks *et al.* 1999 for a discussion of the complex relationships between new technology and democratic reinvention.)

The last part of this chapter briefly explores the policy process and democratic renewal surrounding the uptake of CCTV. It utilises aspects of the theoretical framework put forward by Bellamy and Taylor (1998) and Horrocks *et al.* (1999). In particular, it addresses the question of whether CCTV diffusion is illustrative of a managed topdown process or the result of a more consumerist response to the demands of the general public (a more thorough analysis can be found in Webster 1999).

A 'populist' approach to the democratic policy process would suggest that ICT capabilities are exploited by the existing democratic institutions to enhance the capacity of political and bureaucratic elites to manage democracy and legitimate government activity. In this perspective, a central theme of the management of politics and the policy process is the use of mass marketing techniques such as market research, opinion polls and referenda to represent popular consent for policy and in demonstrating demand for services. In the case of CCTV, it is very apparent that its packaging and marketing has been of fundamental importance in shaping favourable public opinion by projecting the need for increased surveillance. This perspective argues that public information becomes 'commodified' through the increased use of performance indicators and customer satisfaction surveys. Consequently, we are likely to see the shaping, customising and polished packaging of information relating to the performance of services, as well as customers' and citizens' preferences and opinions on service delivery. Information and statistics, such as those used earlier in this chapter (Table 8.1 and Figure 8.1) showing public support for CCTV and its performance achievements, illustrate this point well. Citizens in the populist perspective are passive recipients of policy as determined by policy experts and political elites. Their main role in the policy process is to offer opinions to market researchers. This perspective places considerable emphasis on the management of political communication, which becomes one of the central processes in the public policy process. The emphasis on political elites suggests that the capabilities of new technologies are being utilised to serve the interests of the most powerful actors in the policy process, and that the application of CCTV is being shaped by organisations diffusing the technology to reinforce existing power structures in the policy process and within society more widely.

A more 'consumerist' approach would see policy as shaped to meet the demands of citizens, with the main focus being inclusivity in the policy process and not the legitimacy of the process itself. The consumer democracy perspective argues that individual interests are protected only if the individual has the means to protect them, hence the provision of vast amounts of information about the performance of public services and the increased use of opinion polls and customer satisfaction surveys to gauge public opinion. The key role of the citizen in the public policy process in a consumer democracy is to express and register consumer preferences through market research techniques, which can then be used to shape public policy and the delivery of public services. It is a model, therefore, that sees the individual as active, competent and rational in the making of choices and in the expression of preferences. Citizens become 'stakeholders' in the delivery of service, as improved service provision can be realised only if they concede large quantities of personal data about themselves and their behaviour to the 'informated' state. In the case of CCTV, information about citizens is collected as they go about their daily business. Images can be collected and stored for future reference, such as upcoming investigations and prosecutions. The importance of the new democratic consumerism lies in the fact that the 'consumption nexus' (Bellamy and Taylor 1998) delivers more than just improvements in the efficiency and effectiveness of public services. It is significant in that it joins the need for improved service delivery with a desire to make government responsive and accountable to popular influence.

The material put forward in this chapter suggests that CCTV is a very populist solution to the problems of crime, a straightforward example of politicians providing the service that consumers demand. Those questions raised earlier about the ability of CCTV actually to reduce crime, its impact on human behaviour, the potential threats to civil liberties and the lack of public discourse, imply that CCTV is a symbolic tool that does more to show politicians being responsive to citizens than tackling the complex problems surrounding crime. If this is the case, then it does not actually matter if CCTV is unproven or that it may have undesirable consequences. What is most important is that political reflexivity is realised. This is achieved through a highly managed policy and political process, where public opinion is shaped through agenda setting and information shaping, and critics are marginalised. What this also suggests is that the public policy process operates not necessarily in the public's interest but in the interest of those dominant in society. This is not to suggest a conspiracy managed by the state and against the citizen, rather a 'mobilisation of bias' in favour of CCTV.

The nature of the policy processes surrounding the provision of CCTV and the impact of the technology itself has led to an impoverished manifestation of citizenship. Citizens have a diminished role in the policy process. Where previously they may have participated in public debate and policy consultation, their role is now limited to expressing preferences and opinion about public service. Thus, although the policy process has the appearance of being a two-way process, reducing citizen participation to the expression of service preferences signals a very limited level of citizen involvement in democratic practice.

Conclusion

From the evidence put forward in this chapter, it is clear that citizens are increasingly being watched by CCTV surveillance cameras and that the diffusion and sophistication of CCTV is set to continue. It is also clear that citizens willingly encourage the surveillance of their own movements in return for other perceived benefits, in particular personal safety and reduced crime. The question remains, however, whether we fully understand the policy processes that are leading us to a situation where state surveillance of citizens is the norm. Clearly in the case of CCTV, we are witnessing the emergence of a more managed form of democracy distinct from the traditional, consultative, rational policy process. For example, the importance of packaging strategies highlights the evolution away from traditional parliamentary discourse as the main focus of democratic debate, to a democracy where the packaging and marketing of public policy play a central role in gaining support for those democratic institutions that represent citizens, make policy and deliver services.

A central point of this debate is the question of whether citizen demand for CCTV is genuine and arising from a broad understanding of its technological capabilities, or whether it has been created by those with a vested interest in diffusing the technology. The undeniable popularity of CCTV and its (perceived) ability to reduce crime and the FOC must not detract from the fact that its introduction is altering relations between state and society. To date, public acceptance of CCTV is based on a limited and inaccurate understanding of the functions and capabilities of CCTV technology. CCTV itself, however, is not good or bad, rather it is just a 'technological kit' and a tool that must be placed in its human context and understood in its social, political, economic, organisational and policy environments. Its current application, then, is the result of all those forces shaping its diffusion. What is clearly missing from the current policy process is a wider debate on what kinds of control technologies should be regarded as adequate and necessary in a democratic society in which basic freedoms and human rights are respected.

The rapid uptake of CCTV into public places represents a government-driven technological innovation in the 'fight against crime', and a highly managed policy process in which satisfying citizens' expectations is central to the legitimation of policy and the delivery of services. Undoubtedly, then, the introduction and diffusion of new ICTs in democratic settings is closely interrelated to the emergence of new democratic practices and procedures. Moreover, the emergence of these new democratic and policy processes, illustrated here through the provision of CCTV, is likely to be a feature of governance in the Information Age.

Part III

Digital democracy and civil society

9 Transparency through technology: the internet and political parties

Paul Nixon and Hans Johansson

Introduction

This chapter examines the use of ICTs by political parties and postulates the changes that may accrue from further developments. It incorporates initial observations from the first stages of an ongoing research project concentrating on an analysis of how political parties make use of new technologies. The project took as its pilot case studies Sweden and Holland. Both of these countries have above-EU average levels of computer ownership. Figures as of January 1998 were: Sweden with 26 PCs[1] per 100 inhabitants and the Netherlands with 29.5 per 100 inhabitants, of which 13.6 and 14.8 per 100 inhabitants, respectively, were for private or non-business use (ISPO 1998). In relation to the latter, 330,000 and 404,400 homes, respectively, had internet access as of the end of 1997 (ibid.).

The research was carried out between October 1997 and March 1998.[2] It was largely based upon a series of semi-structured interviews with relevant party officials. At the time of writing, further research is underway in the UK and Estonia, and it is expected that this will expand to include other nation-states as funding and time allow.

The main themes of investigation that are of special interest to us are changes in party organisation and discipline, communications, voting procedures and the overall notion of discursive democracy. We use this term to describe discussion and interaction between individual citizens that may support more consensual forms of decision making. It implies an engagement or involvement in politics that refutes the notion of a passive consumption of 'top down' delivered political views, in favour of 'bottom up' discursive interaction in which the citizen not only consumes but plays a part in the creation of politics. Citizens are increasingly becoming consumers of, not participants in, the political process. It is almost as if there is a form of false consciousness that pervades the majority of the population who delegate politics to a political elite.[3] As one of the people whom we asked to examine the political parties' web sites for us stated: 'I don't want to make all the decisions. That's why I vote [for] the people who will do it for me.'[4]

In terms of a definition of ICTs, we are using this in the broadest sense, although our main emphasis will be upon net-based technologies. It is important to remember that what we often call new technologies incorporate new ways of utilising existing ones, i.e. digital data transfer. One could attempt to provide a definition of ICTs based on illustrative examples, but there are definitional problems in accurately defining ICTs, as their scope and nature is often flexible and open to diverse interpretation (Paletz 1996: 76). What we get is a snapshot of a situation that has, to continue the analogy, moved on since the picture was shot and developed. Whilst this may present problems from a theoretical point of view, the fuzzy definition of ICTs has some advantage in that it facilitates a multidisciplinary approach and emphasises the importance of empirical research within the area.

The societies of the world are going through major technological, economic, political and social shifts. One of these changes, and one that has had an impact upon many other spheres of life, is the development of new modes of information communication. Transition and change are constant forces in human development, and 'they change the everyday cultural ground – the taken-for-granted background conditions of contemporary social life' (Holmes 1997: 6). It would seem as though the change has accelerated during the last decade and shows no sign of abating. The level of social change within the stereotypical western society (if such a thing exists) is increasing. As Dunsire notes:

> until the nineteenth century the dynamic of social change was relatively slow, the line on the graph hardly moving from the horizontal; but then it began to curve upwards and at the end of the twentieth century is not far from vertical: change is not only frequent but fast. Society is highly volatile.
>
> (Dunsire 1994: 21)

Such changes affect political parties, and the ways in which political parties operate will be conditioned, partially, by the technologies available to them. As time moves on, so does technology and the uses that we make of it. For example, as one commentator put it to us: 'There is no point in us producing a CD detailing our policy, as it is too rigid a format and doesn't allow us to change the information at will, as the net does.'

As the political system, along with the responsibilities it undertakes, general political involvement and participation have developed (Katz 1990), there is a recognition that political parties now play a dominant role in politics and governance within the modern Europe (Richardson 1994: 9). Indeed, one could argue that political parties as institutions can be what actually establish the political system in today's society (Finer 1984: 1) The most democratic states today can be said to have adopted the representative system, though it may be in different shapes. All systems from parliamentarianism in e.g. Sweden and England, through combined systems as in France, to presidentialism in the US, have a certain amount of representation.

In order to discuss and analyse how political parties can be affected by ICTs, we need to take account of the role, function and the need for political parties in society. What is a political party? What is it for? Who is it for? Does the party exist for the representatives, the party machine or the ordinary members? One of the major issues facing the modern political parties is active membership. Whilst membership rates are rising in certain parties, e.g. British Labour, there is perhaps a diminution of active members within that party. The very nature of membership has changed, compounded by the increasing moves away from party politics and towards 'direct actions' (Smith 1997). People also no longer necessarily join political parties in order to campaign but in order to endorse and to associate themselves with a certain value set. Just as the trades unions have shifted from their traditional workplace role and have modernised to become 'whole-life' service providers to their members, political parties are starting to restructure and reorientate themselves. If one looks at the traditional view of the British Conservative Party, one could argue that for many of its members it is in fact more of a social networking opportunity than a political party, their prime reason for joining being to meet 'our type of people'.

Traditionally, the representative system has meant that the people have the possibility to choose between different parties in competition. The political parties aggregate values from the people into the political system, and also have the possibility to adopt their own, existing, policy programmes to meet those value-based requirements of the electorate, expressing public interest and prioritising prospective public policy action. These parties then constitute a parliament, based upon the election results, from which is drawn a government. Hence, in the history of political representation, the political parties, as institutions, are the people's representatives in the political system. This of course raises a number of problems:

1   It neglects the role parties play in shaping public opinion.
2   It neglects the fact that they attempt to lead and not necessarily follow public opinion.
3   It assumes that the representatives actually do as their name suggests and represent all the people. It is clear that they do so in name only. The party system exacerbates this. Parties represent sectional interests. One can, however, identify recent attempts to construct a party along the lines of modernised Volksparteien, or what Kirchheimer (1966) calls 'catch-all parties', allied to the use of ICTs. For example, Smith (1997), building upon the work of Downs, supplies the interpretation of the restructuring of political parties shown in Table 9.1.
4   It also neglects a whole area of political activity that takes place often in more informal settings, such as pressure group meetings, internet discourse, etc. The direct interaction between the two types of discourse, – formal/traditional and informal/emergent – being best characterised as lobbying. The separateness of these two worlds, if indeed they ever were truly separate, has been challenged by the advent of interest groups occupying political territory in those policy areas where political parties have failed to incorporate aggregate values. New forms of collective action have been seen to occur, and it could be argued that combined with the move towards traditional politics as infotainment, a depoliticisation of politics is taking place, particularly amongst the young. The established political parties are still important features in the democratic political system, but there are new channels of discourse that share some but not all of the characteristics of traditional political parties.

There are those who see the internet as playing a pivotal part in the future of party politics, but we have to accept that the internet, like any other technology, has advantages and disadvantages. It can be a tool for good in terms of its communication capabilities, or it can encourage new forms of post-hierarchical control (Loader 1997: 1). As Bill Gates notes: 'it [the net] will draw us together, if that's what we choose, or let us scatter ourselves into a million mediated

Table 9.1 Characteristics of three models of party

Characteristics	Mass Party	Downsian Party	ICT/Leadership Party
Principal goals of politics	Pro/anti social reformation	Control of government satisfy majority opinion	Control of government satisfy majority opinion
Pattern of electoral competition	Complete mobilisation of mass membership	Complete mobilisation of available membership	Centrally directed concentration of campaign resources for best returns
Nature of party work and campaigning	Labour intensive	Labour intensive	Activity concentrated in areas where it is likely to deliver the best result
Relationship between ordinary members and elite	Ostensibly bottom-up, though oligarchy develops	Party is a unified team, large degree of decisional involvement	Membership cedes control of initiative to the leadership
Character of membership	Large and homogeneous	Homogeneous	Membership aspect of party in decline in terms of numbers, interest, skills

Source: Smith 1997

communities' (Gates 1995: 274). The main disadvantage, to date, of using the internet within the public sphere, is access (*Guardian* 16 July 1998), which is a constant theme arising from contributions to this collection. Similarly, there is a monopoly of mass-media power-structures, with little opportunity for challenges to the pervading consensus, which distort political messages and limit the opportunity for discursive democracy. This is particularly the case in Sweden, where the media is very 'noll-åtta'[5] (or Stockholm) centric. There is a lack of widely articulated challenge to this mono-cultural view on Swedish political life (Petersson 1998). Conversely, there is also a problem of the internet user being less able to verify the information that they access (Noble 1997).

Before one gets carried away with the notion of a world built upon digital democracy, it is important to remember that there are many people in the world who do not have the means to access this technology. Those with access to the net, the info rich, could be said to be an elite. As one party's internet campaign officer points out: 'the next [Dutch] election campaign will be a mix of online and off-line stuff, with benefits only for the ones who will obey the rules of the internet', thus implying that those who do not or cannot follow the rules of the internet will miss out. Indeed, this situation could deteriorate: with the developments taking place in the televisual/information interface (as noted by Hague and Loader in Chapter 1) and the continuing repackaging of politics as infotainment, one can begin to perceive a future commodification of politics and political information that may threaten effectively to disenfranchise economically some sections of the community.

Just as with tangible resources, distribution of political information will be stratified and uneven as a result of using the internet as a channel of communication. Levels of access will vary, and whilst those who are net-connected may have better access than some, they may also be denied access to other layers of information in the political sphere. Thus we may find an elite within an elite. We must also remember that the situation that we are describing is one that is, to date, only played out in advanced westernised societies. It is easy to forget that in some parts of the world, political democracy is not based upon the same bedrock of participation in liberal democracy as found in the West. Indeed, we need to remember that 70% of the world's population cannot read, let alone operate a computer. As Loader notes: 'most of the world's population has never made a phone call' (Loader 1998: 16). Habermas' concept of '*mediationsverfahren*' butters no parsnips for them.

Let us now move on to examine the following key themes identified at the outset of the chapter:

- organisation and modes of communication
- discursive democracy
- electronic voting

Organisation and modes of communication

To analyse how the organisational forms of political parties are affected by ICTs, it is necessary to make a distinction between structure and function. Different parts of the organisation have different responsibilities and goals. Political parties can hardly be seen as homogenous bodies. The development of political parties has led to diverse and complex organisational forms. This can be seen in two ways, as outlined below.

Organisation by function or group

The political parties have developed into organisations differentiated by function or section/group. Swedish political parties, for example Socialdemokratiska arbetarepartiet (SAP), usually have a women's party or section, a youth party or section, and so on, which are often semi-autonomous from the central party. These sections do not always share an identical perspective with the central party, which can lead to diversity in norms and values and hence to internal conflicts. In terms of developments towards digital democracy, these conflicts may give rise to a situation where separate control over, for example, web pages can lead to conflicting signals being given to the reader (or net visitor). Thus the centre seeks to maintain control over input.

A further problem for the central party machine is that traditional media, such as television or newspapers, have not always conveyed the message as political parties would have hoped. Political parties have often felt that journalists have reinterpreted the message using two strategies: a) by taking power over the interpretation and b) by changing language to distort the message to their own ends (Petersson 1996: 17). Political parties have seen the onset of digital democracy as an opportunity to by-pass traditional media to get their message across (Larsson 1994), attempting to retain tight control over the communication process. Interestingly, a party representative that we spoke to pointed out that many journalists were actually seeking background information, for their stories, from the party's web site, thus offering the party a further opportunity to influence the way in which their activities were presented in the media. Many of the parties believed that traditional briefings via press conferences were open to misinterpretation by journalists in a way that, perhaps, information gleaned from a web site is not. All the political parties that we spoke to, in both countries, were aware of the potential gains to be made by providing a one-stop information shop or virtual cottage, open twenty-four hours a day, all year round. This was of particular importance during the recent elections in both Sweden and Holland.

One or two parties have been tempted to view the internet as a potential communication vehicle that might replace, at least in part, television and newspapers. Most others have seen it as complementing existing communication outlets, and particularly useful for internal communication via e-mail capabilities. The more progressive parties such as D66, in the Netherlands, are ahead in the race to integrate home pages and e-mail systems into intranet systems in order to improve internal communications. The Christen Democratisch Appel (CDA), for example, created an intranet system for their recent election campaign.

The external face of party use of ICTs is the internet home page. All of the major parties have home pages that the public can access.[6] Political parties are, relatively, new to the realm of internet communication. The sites are, relatively speaking, newly created ones, most parties establishing a net presence only in the last four years. Clearly the party and their officials are on a steep learning curve in terms of web page design. As is perhaps to be expected, political parties lag behind the commercial sector in producing challenging and interesting sites. Parties, where they would give us the information, spent amounts ranging from the equivalent of just £3,000[7] up to sums of over £100,000. As a web site manager commented: 'Opposed to other forms of advertising, the internet is, or at least has the potential to be, cheap. There is a certain reluctance to push forward with net communication because the members and voters aren't ready for it.' He went on to say that he felt that this would change as 'a computer literate generation of children today became the voters and activists of tomorrow'.

We found that whilst money was an important factor in producing well-designed, active web sites, those parties that had a more technologically aware activist base, such as the Miljöpartiet or D66, could often compensate for a shortage of funds and create interesting sites. The number of hits, where recorded, varied from approx. 3,000 to over 35,000 per month.[8] As a party web site manager commented: 'Yes, political parties are spending a lot of time, effort and budget ... but they do not always know how to make the best out of it ... the political parties do not take full advantage of all the possibilities offered to them on the internet.'

We asked a small number of non-net users to examine the political parties' web pages in each country. The overall presentation of their observations combined with our other research is the basis of Tables 9.2 and 9.3

Our preliminary observations based on the research, to date, on political parties' use of internet web pages, led us to conclude that we can detect no great difference between political orientation and the amount of effort put into web site design. There is, however, some slight evidence that left-of-centre parties are more ready to adopt ICTs as part of their communication strategy and to seek to gain a new audience from doing so. Their sites tend to be more innovative and, albeit a subjective judgement, more interesting.

The results were not encouraging for the political parties if, that is, they are hoping to attract new voters via the web pages. The information was seen, paradoxically, as being either too basic or too complex. It was often felt to be fairly visually uninspiring and, it has to be said, sometimes not up to date. It must be said that the Swedish sites were felt to be more visually attractive, more informative and more user friendly than the Dutch ones, although it must be remembered that it is possible to have a site that is visually attractive whilst hiding a lack of substantial content (Hunter 1997). Getting the balance right is difficult, as one party web manager remarked:

> When you are a shoe salesman, you sell shoes, so therefore it goes without saying that your target audience will be people looking for shoes. When you are a political party within a society which is way too complex to perceive, an ideology and the various statements on issues are extremely difficult to put on screen and there is no simple way to create a web appearance. None of the original approaches to the other traditional media will work when applied to the internet.

NetPanel recently found, during interviews with 300 'confirmed' net users in the Netherlands, that 75% felt the net to be the appropriate medium for contact between politicians and the public, but

Table 9.2 Examination of political parties' web pages in the Netherlands

Netherlands	PvdA	CDA	VVD	D66	SP	Groen Links
Clarity	+/–	++	+/–	–	++	—
Public discussion possibilities	+/–	—	+	–	++	–
Foreign languages	–	—	—	—	+	+
Publications/ media	++	++	+/–	+/–	+/–	+
Chatrooms available	—	—	—	+	—	—

Table 9.3 Examination of political parties' web pages in Sweden

Sweden	CP	Mod	SAP	MP	FP	ND
Clarity	+/–	++	+	++	—	++
Public discussion possibilities	—	+/–	++	—	—	–
Foreign languages	–	++	+/–	–	+/–	—
Publications/ media	+	++	++	+/–	–	–
Chatrooms available	—	—	++	—	—	—

Key:
+	there is a reasonable amount of . . .
++	there is a lot of/good quality of . . .
+/–	not good but not bad either
–	there is little sign of/not good quality of . . .
—	the home page does not have at all/or the quality is really bad . . .

only 13% of those asked visited the parties' pages regularly (NetPanel 1997). Whilst the internet has been used to provide fairly general information to the public, this information has been rigorously controlled. The party hierarchy would prefer people to stay 'on message'. This is thus going to increase the importance of central control and party discipline, so necessary to preserve the 'iron law of oligarchy' (Michels 1962) and the leader's autonomy in determining party direction (Dunleavy, 1991). Members of left-of-centre parties, such as the SAP in Sweden and the Socialistische Partij (SP) and Partij van de Arbeid (PvdA), in the Netherlands, both originally workers' parties and now designed to appeal to the progressive middleground, were worried that their grip on the democratic process could be loosened by a move away from solidaristic means of decision making, such as mass meetings, towards individualistic decisions engendered by technological impacts upon the parties' channels of communication. Although, as a representative of one party told our researchers:

> The reality is that politicians have less and less contact with the voters. Our party tries to contact, and organise meetings with, people in real life. We, as a party, will use ICTs where modern communication can help us to do things in a better and more appropriate way. Close contact with people who vote for us, is still very important ... and nothing is going to replace that.

It is perhaps interesting to note the potential benefits that might accrue if there were to be a move away from traditional politics towards a digital, discursive democracy. Such a scenario could, for example, encourage more women to enter into political debate, as the relative anonymity offered by virtual discourse (certainly in terms of gender identification) may engender more confidence that the views that they put forward will be judged on their merit and not on the gender of the person putting them forward. It would seem that there may also be a possible diminution of discrimination on other grounds such as race, age, sexual orientation, etc. Of course, in order for this to occur, there would need to be equality of access to the technology, a situation that does not prevail at the time of writing. A spokesperson for one of the Dutch parties expressed the view that whilst ICTs will change relationships between the public and political parties, those changes will be constrained by unequal levels of access to, and acceptance of, ICTs. Thus, the party will be forced to adopt a twin-track communication strategy for those who use the net and for those who, for whatever reason, do not; for, as a politician commented: 'Those who use the internet [for political information] are a small percentage of the population and they do not represent the thoughts of all. When you ask for opinions on the net the results can be leaning very much to one side.'

Organisation by geographical location

There are different forms of organisation within the party in terms of geographical location, from local levels to central level. ICTs play a larger part where distances between centres are greater, such as in the more remote parts of Sweden or where the weather might affect one's ability to travel easily. Here, one finds that there is an increasing use of video conferencing and other technological applications to try to negate the effects of being on the periphery, allowing, at least in theory, the local party organisation to be at the 'virtual centre' of the party machine. At local level, there is increasing frustration at the centre's top down approach to the use of ICTs as a method of control rather than the device allowing for decentralised use (Tops and Depla 1997: 7). Most of the ICT-focused developments, in the parties that we have studied, have been concentrated on the central party machine, although e-mail is presenting opportunities for increased rapid information exchange. All parties have e-mail systems, but the use that they are put to varies across parties. For example, one party spokesperson indicated that only around 25 per cent of their MPs fully utilised the e-mail facilities offered; the rest preferred the telephone as a means of communicating. The spokesperson of another party pointed out that not all those who had e-mail accounts read them, and that if a message was particularly important, then she would telephone to be sure that they got it!

The use of ICTs generally allowed the organisations in our study to be more effective in terms of time and resources and also to be more flexible in their communication strategy. The advent of databases and their use in mail shots was seen as a great boon for party administrators, as they could easily contact their members or contact potential voters, although there are high start-up costs for equipment and software. There are also significant costs in terms of the maintenance and updating of data to meet changing requirements and needs within a modern party machine. In the future, if members were to be online, then presumably e-mail could replace traditional posting methods and allow the transfer not just of standard documents but also of sound and vision and interactive elements. Whilst production costs might be higher, think of the saving involved in sending 1,000,000 e-mails as against 1,000,000 letters, in postage costs alone.

Databases were also a boon during recent elections, allowing parties in our study to disseminate their message to potential voters. Many parties, viewing the ways in which the British Labour Party swept to power utilising ICTs as a component of their election communication strategy, decided to follow suit and adapt their own campaign strategies in subsequent elections in Sweden and the Netherlands. The use of databases has also allowed parties to narrow-cast their message to target voters in key seats during elections. Letters could be crafted to meet individual policy preferences, as determined by the data held upon individuals. Thus, again, we can see the political parties regaining control over messages previously broadcast by traditional media such as TV, radio and newspapers, and subject to their editorial filters. The use of such data to target any form of political marketing has, however, been viewed sceptically by those concerned about the possible erosion of civil liberties (*Guardian*, 16 July 1998) and, indeed, by the parties themselves, who recognise the possible negative effects of unwanted information or junk mail. To recap, we could argue that centralised control has been seen as the driving force, and the perceived gain for the party, rather than utilising new technologies to decentralise power within the party, thus giving it the potential to develop more organically on a local democratic basis.

Discursive democracy

From the party web sites analysed in our study, there is little evidence of attempts to foster discursive democracy in a digital context. Whilst the internet presents great opportunities for new forms of discourse, it can create problems for existing organisations such as political parties or governments. The dynamics of the internet are such that it is difficult to control or 'police'. As Schalken notes, the use of the internet within the public sphere has been primarily evaluated in terms of: 'efficiency and service delivery not ... democracy or the citizen's participation' (Schalken 1997: 12). Thus, political parties are wary of allowing their web sites to slip from their control.

The main use of web sites for discursive democracy was via chat rooms. Whilst these give the impression of a democratic interchange of ideas, one has to question the value that the party places on its content. The chat rooms are often 'ordinary members' exchanging ideas between themselves, and not a bottom up flow informing the policy makers. The leadership/party officials do engage in discussion via the net, but this tends to be on special occasions that are time limited and, generally, have the leader responding to carefully pre-selected points or questions. As we have shown above, control is becoming a key feature of the use of new technology within parties.

The chat room will often have a moderator who will monitor the discussion and has the power to eject those asking inappropriate or difficult questions (Hunter 1997). Even when a party decides to 'moderate' a chat session and to use the data collected as an element in its decision making, just as with e-mail, the costs of administration and response are high and people may not get the level of contact that they desire at the time that they wish, although some MPs suggested that people were more likely to be able to get into contact with them, and receive a reply, by using e-mail than by using the telephone. This is confirmed by one of the aforementioned people who examined the sites for us. She said that she was frustrated by never being able to contact people by phone. Encouraging people to believe that the new technologies will afford them access to the political parties, also builds an expectation that their personal information requests can be met by the party. Again, this adds to the strain on the resources at the parties' disposal, and party workers can be overloaded.

Our analysis of the parties' web sites leads us to conclude that there are missed opportunities for extending discursive democracy into the digital context. Certainly problems related to access may affect accountability. If the parties adopt a more technologically based notion of discursive democracy i.e. digital democracy, it may be more difficult for the non-wired party member, or citizen, to get an insight, or input, into the parties' work. Therefore an important question should be, not only how to use ICT for discussion and debate, but also, what consequences this might have for transparency and democracy?

Electronic voting

Here it can be useful to make a distinction between the process of democracy and the content of democracy, in discussing whether a political system is democratic or not. Process refers to the values and norms that political processes are built on, whereas content refers to 'necessary correspondence between acts of governance and the wishes with respect to those acts of the persons who are affected' (May 1978). Even though this distinction has its critics (Anckar 1982 and Kimber 1989), it remains useful. ICTs have the potential to change, radically, the democratic system as we know it, when it comes to voting procedures. ICTs available today, used to their full potential, afford the possibility to cast one's vote in all instances, including internal party votes. Indeed, this potential is being partially realised, in, for example, Switzerland. How political parties could be affected by ICTs in the area of electronic voting, as an expression of digital democracy, can be viewed in two ways. First, electronic voting could be used within existing party structures, both geographical and sectoral, replacing the ballot paper but still taking place at centrally controlled venues. Second, it could be used to facilitate direct democracy as a challenge to the system of representation through, for example, an increasing reliance on electronic referenda. This means that it would be possible to let the people vote on a day-to-day basis from their homes or other suitable locations.

By creating representative bodies within the organisation, the parties, particularly the members, are doubly dependent upon the individual representative. One of the major effects of ICTs on political parties may be the challenge to the existing representative system. If representatives can be seen as aggregating values, then they can be challenged by the introduction of ICTs, helping the public to perform the same function. This could be achieved by reshaping the role of our present representatives to become information facilitators for home/work-based public voters in a more, but perhaps still not truly, democratic system. Representatives' roles could be adapted to be information presenters to the public at large, charged with disseminating complex information in an entertaining and interesting way. Central party staff would also need to move much more into a role of information gatherers in order to facilitate this. It will then perhaps also be possible to reform the local levels to work in a larger area than was the case when the organisation was more dependent upon the individual representatives. We could speak of ICTs as being a conduit for aggregating values; then one of the most important elements of the political parties' *raison d'être* could be usurped.

Of course, there are problems relating to the representative and the collective party/cabinet/elite retaining the power in terms of agenda setting. The politicians are likely to be loath to give up their grip on power. Turkeys don't vote for Christmas. If the representative system within the political parties may be challenged, then we could expect changes in the organisation forms when it comes to the numbers of levels within the party and what tasks the different levels will have. If the primary task for political parties is to act as a conduit for aggregating public values and proposing policy based upon this, then what will be their function if the party uses ICTs as a method of aggregating individual values? We could argue that political parties, perhaps first and foremost on the local levels, would have to extend their function as a facilitator and provider of political education, debates and other social activities. This could mean that political parties have to change their role and tasks in society to cope with the use of ICTs.

If, as we have postulated, the use of ICTs as a means to aggregate values is forthcoming, this would mean that the representative system as we know it may well be challenged and, to use a Blairite term, modernised or restructured. This may then also require a consequential change in the organisational form of political parties. Also, the different levels, tasks and functions may change as a result of adopting ICTs, and, at a macro level, the political parties may have to re-evaluate their role within the wider political system

This last thought is in line with the notion of participatory/ discursive democracy facilitated by ICTs. The question is why should there be representatives if we (the people) can vote on a day-to-day basis? This implies that both the political system as a whole and the political parties would have to change, when it comes to the Fukiyama-esque end of representative democracy. Evidence from our research would suggest, however, that political parties see little need for a shift along the spectrum to direct or discursive democracy.

If a fuller version of discursive democracy is to occur, then it will depend on the people's ability to understand political questions and the complexity of possible solutions. (One could ask: do many of our representatives understand complex political questions?) Crucially, they will have to want to understand and then to act upon that understanding in terms of democratic participation. Some thought needs to be given as to whether the public actually wish to be involved in a discursive democracy based upon them having to take decisions and to get involved in discussing and debating issues. Many people are happy to offload their participation to representatives.

Conclusions

This chapter has sought to cast further light on the debate around the use of ICTs by political parties. It has shown that whilst parties are adopting some technologies wholeheartedly (e.g. many parties, including GroenLinks, are seeking to use video conferencing as a way of allowing traditional debate and discussion to continue alongside utilisation of technological advances), there are other technological advances that do not always fit with the needs of a modern party.

The contents and number of web sites used by the parties leads to a recognition that there is a continuing conflict within the parties between central control and local autonomy that is open to constant revision. Whilst the Information Age presents opportunities for local democracy, these are often subsumed by the centralising tendencies of the party machines: the 'true' notion of narrowcasting being overtaken by a desire to have 'personalised broadcasting', with the message being slightly altered to meet individual preferences but the content being rigidly controlled from the centre.

The analysis of the developments noted above raises questions not only about what is possible, but also about willingness to accept and adapt to change. One central question is 'Is there a place for the parties of today in tomorrow's political system?' The answer is an emphatic 'No'. First, the parties must have the willingness to change. This will inevitably lead to a recognition that the role and function of political parties in society must be revised. They must adapt or die. They will need to adapt the ways in which they interact with the public and indeed with their own members. In short, a radical reform of their 'corporate vision' is required. As the technologies develop, they will impact upon the organisational forms of the political parties. Coupled with other changes, this could lead to radically differing political parties to those that we know today.

We have seen that there is a reorientation of political discourse taking place, the move from mass meetings to chat rooms being just one example. As this technologically driven reorientation continues apace, alongside other changes, could we see geographical reconfigurations occurring? As the nation-state in Europe is attacked from both above, by moves towards integration and the possible creation of a European super state, and from below, by politically bounded, counter-integrationary forces such as regional devolution as evidenced in the UK and also in Belgium, one has to question the future of the existence of the nation-state. If one accepts that the nation-state's days are, perhaps, numbered, and one then combines these pressures for change with the potential opportunities that the internet possesses in terms of cross-border/cross-cultural activity, which are particularly relevant to discursive democracy, one is drawn to ask the question 'How long will the organisational structures of political parties be determined on national lines?' Is it not conceivable that post-modern times call for post-modern politics and for postmodern structures of organisation. Are we about to see the demise of nationally based parties such as Svenska Miljöpartiet de Gröna or the UK Green Party, and the advent of pan-European political representation far beyond the *ad hoc* voluntary collaborations we have witnessed to date? The technology exists to facilitate such developments; what is lacking at present is the notion of a pan-European identity, although the EU are making strenuous efforts to address this.

That is not all, however. This change in political parties needs to be matched by a change in public perception about democracy and participation or non-participation in the democratic process. Further to this, the problems of access to the technology and to the democratic process must be addressed. This, of course, is reliant upon the development of a strategy to facilitate this. This would form part of a wider project that must address the old, but newly politically sexy, danger of social exclusion.

As we have noted, if we are to move to a political system where an increasing part of political discourse takes place using ICTs, then the issue of access to that technology becomes crucial. Without the social networks, the technology cannot be used to its full potential. Social exclusion and network poverty need to be tackled, and this cannot be done by the traditional methods of turning back to your local community for support. As a recent DEMOS report (1997) showed, in order to break the cycle of deprivation it is necessary to create networks and to see solutions *outside* one's own community. Obviously this takes resources and training that are not always available within certain communities. What we are in danger of moving to, if we adopt an approach based on technological resources that allow us to be defined as information rich, information poor or information excluded, is a society that openly accepts the hegemony of a ruling elite. The idea of information exclusion is one that feeds on ignorance and despair. If we have a role as academics or commentators, it is to ensure that such exclusion does not go unchallenged.

Notes

1 PC is used here as a generic term for all makes of computer, irrespective of operating system.
2 Thanks are due to Kristel Boer, Niels Coelingh Bennink, Jaqueline van Dijk, Magnus Haak, Andreas Harbom, Taru Jussila and Evanthia Kanellopoulou, who did a great deal of the leg work involved in the collection of this data.
3 For reasons of space we cannot develop this argument here, but a fuller exposition will appear in our future work.
4 Please note that all quotations that are not referenced were made during the course of our interviews to support this research. It should also be noted that in some cases the quotations are as translated from Swedish or Dutch. In other instances, where the quotations were given in English (by non-native speakers), these are quoted verbatim.
5 'Noll åtta' (08) is the phone code for Stockholm and used to signify exclusion from the rest of Sweden. It can also be used as a general term of abuse.
6 The home page addresses are as follows:

Netherlands

PvdA	Partij van de Arbeid	http://www.pvda.nl
CDA	Christen Democratisch Appel	http://www.cda.nl
VVD	Volkspartij voor Vrijheid en Democratie	http://www.vvd.nl
D66	Democraten 66	http://www.d66.nl
SP	Socialistische Partij	http://www.sp.nl
GL	GroenLinks	http://www.groenlinks.nl

Sweden

CP	Centerpartiet	http://www.centrepartiet.se
Mod	Moderaterna	http://www.moderat.se
SAP	Socialdemokraterna	http://www.sap.se
MP	Miljöpartiet	http://www.mp.se
FP	Folkpartiet Liberalerna	http://www.folkpartiet.se
ND	Ny Demokrati	http://www.nydemokrati.se

7 In some cases these costings reflected only payments to other agencies and took no account of staff time etc.
8 We cannot be sure of the use those visitors make of the site, how satisfied they are or whether they are repeat visitors.

10 Virtual sounding boards: how deliberative is online political discussion?

Anthony G. Wilhelm

Cyberspace represents another place in which people can communicate politically. Through new venues, people can engage in many sorts of political activity, such as joining interest groups, voting in elections, or participating in political forums. Habermas (1996) suggests that civil society acts as a 'sounding board' for the articulation of political issues to be addressed by government. Thus, those people who discuss political issues in cyberspace can ostensibly raise concerns and express ways of addressing these problems. Of course, political forums ought also to be deliberative, whether they be in cyberspace or face-to-face, since substantive messages must be exchanged in order for the political themes developed in civil society to be translated into items for collective action. The question for empirical research is: how useful are these virtual sounding boards in enabling deliberation in the public sphere? As a corollary to this question, what are the appropriate conditions for enhancing deliberation, so that these forums can more effectively inform and influence the policy process?

Whilst many scholars and practitioners have been swept up in the euphoria surrounding the ubiquitous deployment of teletechnologies, particularly broadband computer networks, it remains to be seen how useful political forums on these networks will be for setting agendas, making public decisions, negotiating differences and arriving at hard-fought compromises (for a teledemocracy literature review, see Dutton 1992). Whilst diversity of voices and universal service are championed as hallmarks of the public interest in US telecommunications policy (Commission on Freedom of the Press 1947), the argument is proffered that these are not sufficient conditions for enabling the articulation of interpersonal, social or political issues and concerns. These discussions must also be deliberative. After all, promoting a diversity of voices, whilst imperative, does not *eo ipso* guarantee deliberation, negotiation and the contestation of view-points (Huckfeldt and Sprague 1995); nor is universal access to these forums sufficient for realising a discursive, democratic polity. Whilst many proponents of teledemocracy anticipate the arrival of ubiquitous, broadband access to the home as the *sine qua non* of democratic reinvigoration, this indicator will not shed much light on the quality of political discourse or the propensity of participants to deliberate to arrive at their goals and objectives. As Benedikt (1991) underscores, it is important to know what may usefully be done in cyberspace before deciding on its viability as a medium for setting political agendas. Whilst the cork has been popped, the froth must settle before the quality of the product can be judged.

This chapter will proceed along the following lines. First, a theoretical framework is put forth in which to understand the features of the virtual public sphere. Deliberation or critical-rational reflection is understood to be a necessary condition of salutary political conversation, without which teledemocracy is as useful as a three-legged chair. Second, a content analysis will be conducted of a sample of political newsgroups to provide empirical validation for the deliberativeness of these new political spaces. Finally, the implications of these findings will be discussed in relation to the overall promise of teledemocracy.

Characteristics of virtual public spheres

What are the characteristics of the public sphere that influence the political potential of this new medium? Clarifying the formal and substantive characteristics of virtual political public spheres allows one to discuss analytically and to test empirically each feature of these novel sounding boards. There are at least five aspects of this space (see Table 10.1), and each characteristic merits proper attention to shed light on the extent to which these venues can provide new avenues for democratic praxis. Whilst this chapter will address only one of these features – deliberation – in depth, the other variables will now be discussed briefly as they affect deliberation.

At the heart of the concept of the political public sphere is its topography, that is to say, the places or spaces in which persons come together to discuss issues, form opinions or plan action. Schneider (1996) calls this space 'the conversational arena', the forums in which space unfolds and new conversations and political discussions can run their course. With respect to topography, an important issue relates to how computer-mediated communication

Table 10.1 Features of the virtual political public sphere

Topography	Places or spaces in which persons come together to discuss issues, form opinions and plan action
Topicality	The content of discussions or the topics that arise
Inclusiveness	Notion that everybody has the opportunity to deliberate on policy issues
Design	The architecture of the network developed to facilitate/inhibit deliberative discussion
Deliberation	Subjecting one's opinions to public scrutiny for validation

(CMC) constitutes people. Whilst many communication researchers suggest that anonymity may liberate the individual and equalise participation in a forum where power is otherwise asymmetrically distributed, others argue that the individual's isolation coupled with invisible surveillance and hierarchical observation from the outside may lead to the veritable incarceration of the user (Kiesler and Sproull 1992). A useful model developed by Spears and Lea (1994), called SIDE (Social Identity and Deindividuation), describes the salient identity present in CMC (e.g. personal or group identity) and its contextual features (e.g. anonymity of in-group or identifying with an in-group). Thus the model reveals the importance of self-categorisation and context-dependence to a proper understanding of cognitive effects. The ramifications for online political debate are important, since this model undermines any reified notions of CMC effects. As the authors argue, 'there are unlikely to be universal effects of CMC because these will be determined as much by social context, the content of identities, and the nature of social relations' (Spears and Lea 1994: 452–3).

The second characteristic of the political public sphere is the content of the dialogue or the topics that are discussed, a feature referred to as topicality. When Habermas portrays civil society as a sounding board, he means in part that it is the public sphere whence ideas, concerns and topics arise, issues which citizens believe need to be addressed by government. The notion of diversity of ideas is critical to an understanding of deliberation, because varying and conflicting views ought to be made available for public consideration. Privileging diversity has been part and parcel of US telecommunications policy, at least since the 1947 Commission on

Freedom of the Press, and its classic statement comes from the Federal Communications Commission's 1949 report explicating the Fairness Doctrine (Kahn 1973). This chapter makes the point that the removal of obstacles to the free flow of ideas is a necessary but insufficient condition for achieving a deliberative political dialogue, whether it be face-to-face or virtual. Intersubjective agreement is not determined solely by the number of ideas that can be vocalised, broadcast or netcast. Whilst the internet may be a potent medium for self-expression, it remains to be seen how effective it will be for collective action. Indeed, the public often becomes awash in words in the absence of editing, filtering and facilitation, not to mention the virtues of listening to and co-operating with others so as to articulate issues to officeholders (Shenk 1997).

In a democratic society, opinion formation and decision making are thought to be legitimating when they represent the will of the people, typically defined as the considered judgement not of a clique or elite group but of all the people who are affected by a policy. In short, democracy means inclusiveness, ensuring that everybody has the opportunity to deliberate on policy issues. In the realm of telecommunications policy, this notion of inclusiveness is captured by the principle of universal service. As Pool suggests, 'from its earliest days, the Bell System's goal and expectation was that telephone service should ultimately be available to everyone in the nation' (1984: 115). In the wake of the Telecommunications Act of 1996 (in particular, Sections 254 and 706), universal service in the USA is subject to an evolving definition as technologies advance. A problem with this new definition, as Sheekey suggests, is that 'market demands and consumer preferences, rather than governmental regulations, will dictate who receives digital information, and at what cost' (1997: 42).

By many accounts, widespread access to advanced telecommunications services, such as electronic mail, will lead to a reinvigoration of democracy. This causal story of ubiquitous access to technology leading to an expanded interest in political matters on the part of the public is accepted, almost with blind faith, although there is scant empirical evidence to support such a lofty claim. Whether it be popular accounts of teledemocracy (Dyson 1997; Katz 1997) or more academic works (Groper 1996), a body of thought is emerging on this matter that mistakes the effect for the cause. Rather than seeing advanced teletechnologies as the amplification of the voices of the socio-economically advantaged and the resource rich (Wilhelm 1997), these writers tend to view technology as the great equaliser, possessing magical powers that can wake up a somnambulistic democracy. This view runs counter to virtually all of the scientific research in the area of political participation, which reveals that the differential availability of resources, including time, skills and money, largely explains who engages in civic and political life (Verba *et al.* 1995).

The fourth general feature of the public sphere is the design or architecture that is developed in order to facilitate discussion. As Guthrie and Dutton (1992) suggest, the design of a network entails a prior policy commitment to the sorts of interactions decision makers want to take place. The design modes arrived at via market and social forces regarding bandwidth issues (Negroponte 1995), cost structure (MacKie-Mason and Varian 1995), user interface concerns, technology architecture and 'rules of order' (Dutton 1996), all told, affect the extent to which content can be delivered, end-users can be information producers and less inhibited yet orderly speech can predominate online. On the issue of architecture, for example, Burgelman (1994) argues that many new distribution media enable consultation but do not allow conversation whereby one can exchange individually stored information, such as e-mail. For example, cable and satellite television as currently arranged may allow the user to request movie selections or see different angles of the baseball field, but they are not interactive in allowing users to be producers of content and to exchange e-mail messages. The design of these teletechnologies seems to be more amenable to plebiscitary democracy, where the individual need only register her preferences, than to a mode of democracy in which conversation, deliberation and critical–rational reflection are integral components.

Finally, deliberation entails subjecting one's opinions to the light of day for validation, in other words, to debate, discussion and persuasion. Private thoughts or isolated activities do not meet the threshold of publicness because they are not exposed to the scrutiny of others. This conception of testing one's ideas in public cuts against the grain of the body of literature in which the public interest is obtained by aggregating individual preferences (Petracca 1991). To repeat, whether it be the early QUBE experiments or the latest beta-tests for interactive services, customer choices are limited to registering preferences on a keypad, a process that falls short of democratic deliberation in which participants validate their ideas against those of their peers in the public square (Elshtain 1982).

Clearly, the five features of the political public sphere enumerated in this section are inextricably linked. Network design is obviously critical to interactivity as well as to the regulation of speech (e.g. netiquette), and both of these features are requisite to deliberation. Universal accessibility to forums is also necessary to provide a diversity of viewpoints and to ensure that the voices of the subaltern are acknowledged, whilst this does not guarantee a substantive discussion, as has been pointed out. Understanding the new topography of cyberspace is important in determining how time and space as traditional components of a political discussion (i.e. carried on in a chamber or townhall, in a face-to-face manner, usually with certain time limitations) are subverted within Taylor and Saarinen's (1994) 'mediatrix', a place–event in which anonymity, isolation and asynchronism become familiar landmarks of political life. Finally, online content is an important issue that overlaps with deliberation, since restrictions on and regulation of internet content may have lasting effects on political speech. The 1996 Communications Decency Act in the USA, for example, proscribed the transmission of indecent and obscene speech. In the aftermath of its passage, salutary political content, such as information on AIDS awareness and prevention, safer sex practices, as well as gay and lesbian issues, has in some instances been proscribed (American Civil Liberties Union 1996). The empirical findings will require us to revisit the features of virtual public spaces in the conclusion of this chapter, in suggesting ways in which any or all of them may be refined to enhance democratic deliberation.

Exploratory questions

According to Fishkin (1995), the contemporary political scene is characterised by democracy without much deliberation. With the subversion of deliberative democracy (McChesney 1997), the interests represented by various public spheres may lack the consideration and authority that are needed to affect substantively the policy agenda. As Barber argues, 'talk radio and scream television have already depreciated our political currency, and new technologies are as likely to reinforce as to impede the trend if not subjected to the test of deliberative competence' (1995: 270). But what exactly is deliberation? Fishkin (1992) tells us that there are three conditions that make face-to-face deliberation possible:

1 political messages of substance can be exchanged at length;
2 there is opportunity to reflect on these messages as well as for ongoing debate and reflection; and

3   the messages can be processed interactively, with opinions being tested against rival arguments.

Applied to Usenet political forums, one might expect that these three conditions could be readily met. One might even suppose that Usenet is ideally suited to deliberative exchange, since the asynchronous and virtual nature of the technology allows for reflection, whilst its software enables participants to respond to postings and to incorporate their remarks effortlessly into an ongoing thread.

Whilst on the face of it Usenet may appear to facilitate deliberative speech, it is necessary to explore empirically the incidence of considered, critical–rational conversation on its political forums. The interdisciplinary literature on CMC effects, empirical evidence from past and present teledemocratic experiments, and normative theorising provide a rich set of questions for exploration. The following queries are posed to clarify the degree to which discussion migrating to new communication networks displays or approximates any or all of the salutary characteristics of deliberation as described by theorists and practitioners.

The first research question to be addressed is: to what extent do participants of virtual political groups solely provide ideas and information versus seeking information from other forum members? There are hundreds of postings on Usenet political newsgroups every day, but, as has been suggested, the quantity of postings does not guarantee equal participation (Schneider 1996) or vigorous exchange of opinion. It is vital to discern how often these postings are aimed at seeking out, acquiring, filtering and exchanging information to increase awareness and understanding. According to Neuman (1991), in seeking information, people gather only what is necessary to make reasonable decisions on issues. If there are considerably more postings that begin and end with providing and seeking information, then it is hard to imagine reciprocal acts occurring in which participants in a political discussion articulate their interests through talking, sharing ideas and negotiating differences. Political talk then involves receiving as well as expressing, in other words, acknowledging information or ideas that complement one's own ideas and thoughts (Arendt 1977).

The second research question is: to what extent do participants of political groups exchange opinions as well as incorporate and respond to others' viewpoints? As teledemocratic experiments illustrate, there is a tendency to substitute deliberative political discussion with 'push button' or plebiscitary democracy, in which individuals

register their preferences on issues without exchanging ideas or interacting with others (Arterton 1987). In effect, this portrait of direct
democracy values individuals as information providers, in registering
their preferences, and discounts interaction and conversation with
other citizens. Whilst the first question addresses the extent to which
participants are using newsgroups simply to amplify their own views,
the second question begins to discern the extent to which political
newsgroups are genuinely interactive. As Fishkin puts it:

> when arguments offered by some participant go unanswered by
> others, when information that would be required to understand
> the force of a claim is absent, or when some citizens are unwilling
> or unable to weigh some of the arguments in the debate, then
> the process is less deliberative because it is incomplete.
>
> (Fishkin 1995: 41)

The third query is: to what extent is there in-group homogeneity
of political opinion on Usenet newsgroups? Research shows that
people prefer to form groups among those with whom they agree,
a phenomenon known as homophily (Huckfeldt and Sprague 1995).
In terms of the opinions that are fostered in these groups, social
psychology research shows that in-group favouritism exists in which
group members are less judgeable than out-group members (Yzerbyt
et al. 1995). In addition, out-group members are perceived as more
homogeneous in their traits and behaviour than in-group members.
Homogeneity has been defined differently depending on exactly
what researchers are attempting to identify. In this case, homogeneity
is defined as the extent to which individual messages adhere to a
certain political affiliation, defined as endorsing or supporting a political candidate, platform, issue or ideology. In a study of political
identity within British political parties, Kelly (1989) found that homogeneity was correlated with increased salience of key political
objectives, such as promoting unity and strength. It will be interesting to know whether Kelly's findings are applicable on Usenet
groups with well-defined agendas.

To illustrate this point, the content analysis on which this chapter
is based was conducted in October 1996, during the presidential
campaign homestretch in the USA. At this time there were many
postings on various aspects of the candidates' character, position on
issues and so forth but, exchanges of opinion between messengers
with diverse viewpoints occurred infrequently. The newsgroup
alt.politics.liberation, for example, included scant criticism of the

Libertarian presidential candidate, Harry Browne, or of the party platform. Almost every message either strongly affirmed or at least indirectly affiliated itself with the Libertarian agenda (i.e. either its presidential candidate or party platform). In so doing, forum participants demonstrated strong in-group homogeneity. To make educated choices among political candidates, however, citizens probably need to canvass different viewpoints and assess and re-evaluate their own position based on new information. This presupposes a political forum with internal imperatives for critique and discourse. Participating in forums where in-group identity is strong may truncate such an exercise.

The final question relates to the critical–rational dimension of newsgroup political discussions: to what extent are substantive, practical questions debated rationally in contradistinction to *ad hominem* argumentation not susceptible to criticism and grounding? This is a challenging question, since messages presenting a rational argument in some cases may not easily be differentiated from arguments in which assertions are not validated. To clarify this issue, rationality was assessed in the light of Habermas' (1984) distinction among the semantic content of these expressions, their conditions of validity and the reasons for the truth of statements or for the effectiveness of actions. In other words, the rationality of an assertion depends on the reliability of the knowledge embedded in it. Knowledge is reliable to the extent that it can be defended against criticism. Forum participants can supply reasons in defence of a certain proposition, and, to the extent that they are recognised as reasons, members can orient their actions to intersubjectively recognised validity claims. In the absence of reasons or intersubjectively recognised validity claims, it is unlikely that claims will be adjudicated. To illuminate this point, one forum that was examined, alt.politics.white-power, included a range of discussion describing the physical features of Africans, some comments reminiscent of phrenological arguments from the nineteenth century. In other words, its semantic content was dissonant, unmoored to contemporary language norms. Whilst this fact alone does not discount its potential validity, forum participants seldom advanced arguments or reasons to support their assertions, which means that the truth of their statements was not defended and made accessible to the scrutiny of the larger public.

Data and methods

Content analysis was chosen as the appropriate methodology to address these questions. Since the deliberativeness of online political communication is really about the substantive components of messages as well as about reciprocity between messengers (also judged in this instance exclusively by examining the relationship between messages), content analysis was determined to be the tool most amenable to discoveries about the four questions enumerated in the previous section concerning: information seeking, interactivity of opinion, homogeneity and rationality. Content analysis is 'a research technique for making inferences by systematically and objectively identifying specified characteristics within a text' (Stone *et al.* 1966). This methodology has been used to understand group behaviour (Sproull and Faraj 1995) but not to explore the deliberativeness of self-identified political forums.

There are two principal advantages of using content analysis as the appropriate methodology for this study. First, as explained by Krippendorff (1980), content analysis is a study of data as they appear in a context, enabling one to examine extant texts. Political postings and the threads of discourse in which they are embedded comprise a defined context or horizon from which a discussion can be evaluated. It is not necessary to know who the participants are, from what walk of life they come or with what political parties they are affiliated, to paint a compelling portrait of the deliberativeness of these discussions. As Sproull and Faraj ascertain in their study of Usenet communities, 'the benefits provided by electronic groups often extend beyond the direct participants when members act as conduits of information to people outside the group' (1995: 75). This generalization was arrived at not by asking messengers what they do with the information they receive via Usenet postings, but rather from the very content (or context) of the messages themselves. Of course, it is exceedingly difficult from content-analysing messages to judge, say, the amount of time participants spend critically reflecting on other postings, either by themselves or with family and friends. This is a limitation. But as Spears and Lea argue, regarding a message as 'what is made salient and meaningful in the context' rather than simply what is transmitted or omitted provides us with a 'powerful and flexible theoretical tool for understanding the wide-ranging effects of CMC' (1994: 452).

Second, compared with interviews or ethnographic study, content analysis usually 'yields unobtrusive measures in which neither the sender nor the receiver of the message is aware that it is being analyzed' (Weber 1990: 10). Questioning respondents or having them fill out surveys, from the perspective of content analysis, is about creating new texts, ones that are sometimes biased by the interests of researchers and the pressure felt by interviewees to supply acceptable responses. For example, a questionnaire of political attitudes may yield what are called socially acceptable responses. Respondents may exaggerate the extent to which they participate politically and deliberate on party platforms. Since participants in political forums are unaware that their messages are being studied, they are not affected by the glare of researchers and their instruments.

At the initial stage of this study, it was necessary to determine the unit of analysis to arrive at a sample frame. Since information was sought primarily on the makeup of messages, the single posting was the principal unit of analysis. Thus, a sufficient number of messages was included in the sample to generalise their characteristics (N = 500). In addition to the individual posting, message strings were analysed, such as the relationship between messages, newsgroup homogeneity and the number of threads. Thus, the newsgroup became the appropriate unit of analysis (N = 10). In order to gauge this information, a sample of political newsgroups was selected, an appropriate number to assure that a variety of forums was analysed but not too many to be unnecessarily burdensome to coders. These messages were drawn from Usenet political newsgroups as well as from America Online's (AOL) 'Washington Connection'. A commercial ISP was examined for two reasons: to ascertain how deliberative its forums were relative to the categories described in the previous section; and to determine how these discussions differed, if at all, from Usenet political forums. When the content analysis was conducted, in October 1996, there were fifty-seven newsgroups self-described as political and fourteen discussion groups on 'Washington Connection' (see Appendix to this chapter). Although many Usenet newsgroups deal with political themes, the study was limited to those forums whose addresses reflect political content and objectives.

From each newsgroup, an identical number of messages was selected for content analysis over roughly the same period of time. To be more specific, the following procedure was observed to arrive at a random sample of messages for analysis:

1   an equal number of consecutively posted messages were downloaded from ten newsgroups chosen at random (six from Usenet newsgroups and four from AOL);

2   to be confident that the sample represents the universe of messages posted to political forums, a sample of 500 messages was needed to ensure a satisfactory confidence interval (± 4.4 per cent);

3   therefore, fifty messages were selected from ten groups, selected at random, for a total of 500 messages;

4   a roughly equal time period was randomly selected to capture continuity in themes across lists;

5   to capture threads within groups, the fifty messages from each group were consecutive. A randomly selected day and time was chosen, and messages were downloaded from each group covering approximately the same period of time.

To ensure that the findings were reliable, 10 per cent of the messages were coded by an independent coder, once the appropriate units and categories had been developed and the coders were trained. The coefficient of reliability was found to be 0.84, demonstrating a high degree of interjudge consistency (Janda 1978; Krippendorff 1980).

Content categories

The concept categories were developed to operationalise the questions posed in the previous section. It was important to ensure that the content dictionary categories actually shed light on the questions that this study aims to address. In other words, the issue of face validity was addressed by matching content definitions with the questions to be clarified, as is shown in Table 10.2. The first research question, for example, asks the extent to which participants provide ideas and information versus information seeking. This was measured through two specific content categories. First, the category PROVIDE was developed to analyse messages in terms of whether they involve solely the provision of information or content to the forum. Any message that involves interactivity or query is coded accordingly (e.g. as INCORP or REPLY). Of course, Usenet technology includes store and forward software where a user typically posts a follow-up article to the entire newsgroup. Rather than coding such a message as being interactive, however, the content itself was examined. If the message makes no reference to another posting and does not make queries seeking information, then it is coded as PROVIDE. The other category used to clarify this question is called SEEK, which describes only those messages that involve instances of information seeking, usually in the form of queries to other forum members.

Rather than coding these two categories in terms of preponderance (e.g. determining whether a message is more about providing information or more about seeking information), a message that included any tangible evidence of information seeking behaviour was coded as SEEK. A message may include a long diatribe on a particular political issue, but if there is at least one sentence or instance of inquiry, then it is labelled as SEEK rather than PROVIDE. A third category is a special instance of either of the first two categories in which a message provides the spark for a discussion train, known as a thread. This category is referred to as SEED, since it includes only those messages that are original, that is, preceding subsequent reply messages in time.

The second set of categories moves us into the realm of genuine reciprocity. INCORP is a category that operationalises whether messages include opinions or ideas drawn from information sources other than postings within the newsgroup, either from expert information providers or other citizens. INCORP may also be coded as SEEK, but the reverse cannot be true. REPLY refers to a message that is a response or reply to another message previously posted. Unlike INCORP, in which a posting may include information from other sources not participating in the political newsgroup in question, REPLY includes only those messages that are direct responses to previous postings.

The third question is addressed by the content category, HOMOGE-NOUS, which is a measurement of the extent of political affiliation that postings demonstrate. Political affiliation here means evidence of messages adhering to key political objectives, such as solidarity toward a political candidate, party platform, issue or ideology. Coders assessed this affiliation based on the overall tone of the message, and ranked the extent of affiliation on an interval scale (4 = strong affiliation; 3 = weak/moderate affiliation; 2 = no affiliation; 1 = weak/moderate disaffiliation; 0 = strong disaffiliation). These results were summed across a newsgroup and then averaged so that a newsgroup that demonstrates strong homogeneity of opinion, such as alt.politics.libertarian, for example, would score near a 4, whilst a political forum where there was high disaffiliation would obviously score substantially lower.

Evaluating a message based on its overall relationship with a dominant position might seem to beg the question of what is the affiliation of each message. This two-stage approach canvasses the newsgroup for dominant themes, ideologies or agendas, however, and then codes individual messages as they relate to these prevailing viewpoints. By

Table 10.2 Political messages content dictionary categories

Tag	Full name and definition	Face validity
provide	PROVIDE: a message that is solely providing information from other participants in the form of facts, opinions and the like	Q#1
seek	SEEK: a message that includes evidence of information seeking in the form of queries, open-ended remarks and the like	Q#1
seed	SEED: a message that plants a seed for discussion, usually providing the groundwork for a topic, always the first in a series of reply messages	Q#1
incorp	INCORPORATE ideas drawn from others, whether they be experts or other citizens but *not* those who are participants in the exchange in question	Q#2
reply	REPLY: a message that is the response or reply to another message previously posted	Q#2
homogenous	HOMOGENOUS: the extent to which the sum of messages analysed on a single political newsgroup approach strong political affiliation on dominant or prevailing agendas, measured as mean value scored on interval scale of 'extent of political affiliation'	Q#3
validate	VALIDATE: an expression that is subject to criticism and grounding assessed in light of the internal relations between the semantic content of these expressions, their conditions of validity and the reasons (which could be provided, if necessary) for the truth of statements or for the effectiveness of actions	Q#4
novalid	NOVALID: an expression that presents neither conditions of validity nor reasons for the truth of the statement – instead appeals are made largely to personal prejudice, emotion or aesthetic judgement	Q#4
aut	AUTHOR: the mean number of authors posting per day	
length	LENGTH: the mean length of a message, measured as number of words	
message	MESSAGE: the mean number of messages per day	
time	TIME: the mean time length of a thread in days	
thread	THREAD: the mean number of threads per day, a thread being a continuous discussion on a single topic or related topics occurring over a particular period of time	

canvassing dominant threads and in assessing the overall tone of a newsgroup, deductively, dominant positions or prevailing views were identified (if social identity theory is correct on the priority of in-group homogeneity, then an asymmetrical political balance of newsgroup messages should be expected). Then, in an inductive or analytic approach, each message was coded to determine the extent to which it cohered to this dominant position. Whilst this approach is by no means failsafe, it should yield a rough indication of in-group homogeneity.

The fourth research question is answered by the content categories VALIDATE and NOVALID. Habermas attempts to define arguments that are amenable to rational agreement as holding out the premise 'that *in principle* a rationally motivated agreement must always be reachable, where the phrase "in principle" signifies the counter-factual reservation "if argumentation were conducted openly and continued long enough" (1990: 105). Rationality, for Habermas, is assessed 'in light of the internal relations between the semantic content of these expressions, their conditions of validity, and the reasons (which could be provided, if necessary) for the truth of statements or for the effectiveness of actions' (1984: 9). In short, if postings supply reasons or arguments for the validity of their positions, then they provide the groundwork for a rationally motivated agreement to be reached. If valid reasons are not advanced, then subjects, rather than exchanging validity claims, may not be able to find common ground.

The other content categories, the last five in Table 10.2, are self-explanatory. They are critical to understanding how long political conversations persist, how durable discussion threads are and the like. These content categories highlight the lifecycle of discussion threads and suggest incidence of deliberation as a function of time, not just its critical–rational dimension.

Let me provide a sample message and discuss briefly how these content categories would apply to it. The following message was posted to the newsgroup alt.politics.elections in October 1996, shortly before the presidential election:

> Bob Dole has to be the most boring, gray, uncharismatic person ever to run for president of the US. He comes across as tired, bitter and humorless. Good thing he's in between jobs. I wonder how becoming president would affect his character. A grimace would probably assume permanent residency in his face. Not that Clinton is fantastic, mind you, but he seems much more

energetic and compassionate. Electing Dole would be like electing the crabby neighbor down the street.

Clearly, this message exclusively provides information to the newsgroup, primarily concerning the character and personality of the two principal presidential candidates. The author neither makes an enquiry of the newsgroup nor directly responds to another message. Of course, from the context of previous postings, it may be ascertained whether this message is indeed a response to a previous posting. On the face of it, however, this message does not meet the threshold for coding it as interactive or involving an exchange of opinions. Assessing its relationship with the prevailing theme of its thread, involving a sustained critique of Bob Dole's character and personality, reveals a display of strong in-group affiliation *vis-à-vis* an evaluation of Bob Dole's candidacy. Coders scored this message as a 4, which means it demonstrates strong affiliation with the in-group's agenda. In terms of the rationality of the message, it clearly fails Habermas' (1984) test of providing reasons to validate the truth of assertions made about Dole's character and Clinton's personality. These reasons may be latent and may or may not emerge if the author is prompted; for the sake of this coding scheme, however, if reasons are not supplied in the message itself, then its validity is diminished as a statement that would enhance the deliberative process of the newsgroup participants. Thus, it is coded as NOVALID.

Findings/discussion

The first question aimed to clarify the extent to which political discussion in cyberspace involves information seeking, that is, the use of these newsgroups to enquire about political matters. The content analysis reveals that the bulk of political messages primarily provide a text, usually less than 100 words, rather than seeking information from other messengers. As Table 10.3 shows, slightly less than three out of four messages exclusively provided information to the newsgroup, whilst the figure is approximately 30 per cent for those that are information seeking and less than 20 per cent that are seed messages. Clearly, the bulk of newsgroup postings are an expression of ideas and opinions provided to a forum. Only a fairly small percentage of messages actually seek out information on a particular topic. These postings provide a point of departure for a conversation; but if nobody responds to them, then they may well add so much grist to the mill.

Table 10.3 Content analysis results

Content categories	Political newsgroups	AOL's 'Washington Connection'	
PROVIDE	71.2%	67.3%	Q#1
SEEK	27.9%	32.5%	Q#1
SEED	15.7%	18.2%	Q#1
INCORP	52.9%	47.7%	Q#2
REPLY	15.5%	23.1%	Q#2
HOMOGENOUS	$\mu = 3.1$	$\mu = 3.2$	Q#3
VALIDATE	67.8%	75.6%	Q#4
NOVALID	32.2%	24.4%	Q#4
AUT	$\mu = 16.3/\text{day}$	$\mu = 10.3/\text{day}$	
LENGTH	$\mu = 97.3$ words	$\mu = 102.5$ words	
MESSAGE	$\mu = 19.1/\text{day}$	$\mu = 11.3/\text{day}$	
TIME	$\mu = 3.1$ days	$\mu = 4.1$ days	
THREAD	$\mu = 3.7/\text{day}$	$\mu = 2.6/\text{day}$	

The political forum alt.politics.org.cia, for example, was one on which postings by individuals were often long, intricate and involved, yet there was very little questioning of newsgroup participants about particular issues. One messenger posted arcane multipage, multi-series messages on encryption, which may have been informative to a portion of the audience; however, nobody posted a response or posed a question to this gentleman. Whilst it was a diverse forum in terms of the number of issues covered, it rarely hosted interactive exchanges.

The second question asked whether participants in political forums are incorporating the views of others in their ongoing quest for information and conversation. Is there a sense in which the messages present on these forums comprise a series of conversations? Is the knowledge and information transmitted in any way discursive, geared toward co-ordinating action among participants? As Barber informs us, 'strong democracy promotes reciprocal empathy and mutual respect' (1984: 223). Based on this study's limited coding categories, however, online participants are not responding to the views of other group members. Fewer than one out of five messages represents a direct reply to a previous posting, which suggests the notion of an attenuated public sphere (see Table 10.3).

In their study of six Usenet newsgroups, Sproull and Faraj found evidence for substantial social interaction, enough to evoke the metaphor of the 'gathering place' to describe the contours of these social spaces. They suggest that over one-half of the messages that they coded demonstrate social interaction; that is, they induce one or more replies or are themselves replies to previous postings (1995: 69). Whilst this study accords with Sproull and Faraj in viewing virtual public spheres as fulfilling the human need for affiliation, these forums may be more akin to what Schudson (1997) calls 'the sociable model of conversation', oriented toward the pleasure of interacting with others in conversation rather than toward addressing or solving problems. The problem-solving understanding of conversation is one geared towards the articulation of common ends. Data gathered in Table 10.3 do not support the problem-solving mode as the chief characteristic of online political discussion. Indeed, even the social model is an attenuated one when so many of the messages posted on these forums are unrequited.

If a democratic discussion is to be defined at least in part by the quality of the conversation, then the newsgroups analysed in this study are not very deliberative. Rather than listening to others, more often than not persons opposed to a seed message used it to amplify their own views. Perhaps one reason why there are so few responses is that there is no obligation to respond on the part of either latent or active forum participants. That is to say, since messages are not addressed to particular respondents (as, say, a letter would be), there is no imperative to respond on the part of an anonymous addressee. In societies where a right of response is valued (e.g. *le droit de réponse* in France), citizens are 'more than the fraction of a passive, consumer "public"' (Derrida 1992). Where democracy is desired, there must be reciprocity. Reciprocity is unlikely in forums where participants do not feel responsible before other forum members.

With respect to the third question, concerning the extent of group homogeneity, the prevailing view seems to define these forums in terms of 'communities of interest', virtual gathering places in which those people who share a common interest can discuss issues without substantial transaction or logistical costs. This understanding supports the view that individuals tend to seek out those individuals (and affiliations) with whom they agree. As Huckfeldt and Sprague argue:

> groups that are evenly divided in political opinion, or approximately so, must be rare. Asymmetry in the distribution of beliefs within groups is likely to be prevalent, particularly since it is

known that individuals tend to seek out politically like-minded associates.

(1995: 53)

Testing this phenomenon reveals over 70 per cent of messages characterised as homophilic, that is, demonstrating either strong or moderate support for the dominant position on a political topic or candidate. The modal value for the scores was a 4 and the mean score was about 3.2, which means that strong affiliation with dominant themes and agendas was evident (see Table 10.3). Many forums that had a well-defined agenda revealed strong in-group identification, which means that the identity of a newsgroup is critical in understanding the extent to which it can be expected to be homogeneous.

The political forum alt.politics.libertarian was examined to explore the extent to which agreement or homophily exists on this group. If Downs' (1957) model – that persons will want to reduce their information costs by obtaining information from like-minded individuals (e.g. Democrats from other Democrats or the Democratic Party) – is assumed, then one would predict that this forum, dedicated to Libertarian ideology, would include a skewed distribution of viewpoints. This hypothesis was validated by content analysing the fifty messages on this forum for homogeneity of political positions. Over 90 per cent of the messages to which a political affiliation could be ascribed were Libertarian or were supportive of some Libertarian tenets. Since the content analysis was conducted one month before the 1996 presidential election, there was considerable traffic lauding Harry Browne, the Libertarian presidential candidate. There was only one criticism of Browne, from a man who believed that his candidacy represented 'a right-wing militia front'. Notwithstanding this fact, the messenger remained committed to the Libertarian platform. The discourse on this forum was overwhelmingly hostile to government and supportive of empowering the individual, as one might expect. Often, government regulation and involvement in society were characterised as 'bone headed' or 'draconian', and these comments were, on the whole, unopposed by lurkers who may not have possessed Libertarian predilections.

The notion that a virtual community entails the organisation of people around a common interest follows from the empirical data. The implications of these findings, however, are far from obvious. In terms of developing issues to be processed by policy/makers, communities of interest may form around issues that, for whatever reason, have yet to generate support in civil or political society. As Habermas points out, many issues that concern not just the problem of distribution but the 'grammar of forms of life' (1987: 391–4) have yet to be adequately addressed by governmental policy, whether it be the issue of individual self-realisation, quality of life or equal rights for all groups. Communities of interest could take on the role of identifying and promoting these issues before government. The downside of in-group homogeneity is that it may become more difficult in an increasingly pluralistic society for new identities to co-exist. As Connolly warns, 'any drive to pluralization can itself become fundamentalized' (1995: xi), suggesting that as individuals continue to find success in affiliating with like-minded souls, their 'drive to pluralization' may make finding common cause with other groups more difficult.

The final question explored the extent to which online political messages are amenable to Habermas' (1984) conception of rational agreement. Of the random sample of messages analysed, as Table 10.3 illustrates, about three out of four provided reasons to justify their statements; the remainder of the postings did not validate or support their statements with arguments. The political forum called alt.politics.white-power included discussions of the size of the lips of Africans as well as other characteristics of minorities that several participants themselves believed crossed the line between reasoned argument and personal prejudice. One participant called the ancient Egyptians 'xenophobic', and a respondent said that his 'descriptions were based on prejudices, not factual reality'. Another participant suggested that there is a 'cephalic index' which shows that the skulls of Africans differ from those of whites. A respondent asked this person if he 'would care to tell us what these alleged distinctive features are and provide some evidence'. Unfortunately, very little validation for these ideas was forthcoming. Notwithstanding the bald assertions made in this particular forum, an overall high degree of critical–rational text was evinced on Usenet and AOL political forums. Perhaps this was in part due to the fact that users had time to compose their messages in relative isolation and anonymity. Unlike face-to-face communication, in which there is often the need to respond expeditiously to other respondents, say, in a townhall discussion, participants in online forums are not burdened to respond immediately to other citizens. They are thus afforded the time and anonymity to craft political messages that can reflect their considered judgement.

In addition to the questions enumerated above, there are important aspects of the durability of threads that are key to understanding online democratic deliberation. The content analysis reveals that a considerable portion of politically oriented messages posted to newsgroups as well as the commercial site, AOL, demonstrate attenuated, episodic and ephemeral social interaction. Only about 20 per cent of messages were actually addressed to other messengers, which suggests that sustained dialogue among all participants on a single topic or line of inquiry is uncommon.

These virtual gathering places are home to an array of overlapping and short-lived threads. Participants come and go, many perhaps lurk or read the posted messages without offering a testimonial. As is clear from Table 10.3, on any given day there are about three separate threads or conversations occurring via political newsgroups or AOL's 'Washington Connection'. Each thread lasts about three days on the newsgroups and about four days on the commercial network. Perhaps the threads last longer on America Online because there are slightly fewer messages posted per day. Whilst Metcalfe's law suggests that the value of a network increases by the square of its users, the ephemeral nature of many threads is inauspicious for the formation and continuation of deliberation on a range of policy issues, since it is uncertain whether such short-lived conversations can ultimately have an impact on what is put on the policy agenda. Although Metcalfe's law is often used to defend universal service policies in which a network's value increases as the number of subscribers increases, the law is an insufficient validation for such a policy. Whilst it may indeed be true that the size of the potential participant pool is often inversely related to the quality of discussion that can be achieved (Dennis and Valacich 1993), many forums comprise postings that are primarily information providing, a phenomenon that does not require that users exchange viewpoints and consider other opinions. Perhaps Rheingold (1993) put it best when he suggested that although people might appear to be 'conversation addicts', many of these gathering places seem to reflect much more talking than listening. It may be perfectly justifiable to subsidise public access to the internet either on the basis of ensuring individual self-expression or safeguarding democracy by creating an informed and educated citizenry; its benefits as a vehicle for collective action, as currently designed, however, may be limited (Dutton 1996).

As is clear from Table 10.3, there are two major differences between AOL forums and Usenet newsgroups, as could be determined by the limited coding categories and relatively small sample sizes. The first is that the AOL forums were significantly smaller than the average Usenet newsgroup. This size difference perhaps translates into a greater likelihood on the part of America Online users to consider the viewpoints of others when they post messages. Since newsgroups can be quite large, with numerous daily postings and a phalanx of threads, it may well be more difficult for users to find a point of entry into a discussion, as opposed to a smaller forum in which fewer messages are more sporadically posted. There is more conversation of a rational–critical nature on AOL as well, which could be attributed in part to the smaller circle of participants as well as to the sense of dialogue that is created by AOL's 'guides', who may contribute to its public relations by promoting forums, greeting members and even contributing to chat rooms, thus creating a kind of potemkin village with respect to political discourse.

Conclusion

The sorts of virtual political forums that were analysed do not provide viable sounding boards for signalling and thematising issues to be processed by the political system. They neither cultivate nor iterate a public opinion that is the considered judgement of persons whose preferences have been contested in the course of a public gathering; at least there is insufficient evidence to support such a salubrious picture of the political public sphere in cyberspace. Critics may suggest that holding actual political engagement up to the standards of democratic theory is unfair, since the way in which people relate to each other will only on rare occasions rival the ideal. It must be underscored, however, that if cyberspace is going to be a venue for identifying, articulating and even solving political problems, then it is necessary to discover how these tasks can be discharged. Evaluating various projects in terms of how they allow participants to solve problems, as well as experimenting with new forum designs, may lead to a clearer picture of the relative merits of these venues for deliberation and critical debate.

Although the drum beat is often heard that liberal democracy is moving towards a more direct form of civic and political participation, in part due to teletechnologies that can enable home-based engagement, a wide gap exists between what can be done, technologically, and what should be done, from a political and ethical point of view. If so-called netizens have not tested their opinions in the light of day, then attenuated political discourse and push-button democracy may well represent the Information Age's high-water mark.

In order to enhance teledemocracy's potential, it is necessary to relate the findings briefly to the other characteristics of the political public sphere in order to suggest several palliatives. The following indicate several possible directions. In terms of the inclusiveness of these forums, universal participation cannot be guaranteed. There will always be people who are unable or unwilling to engage in the sorts of discursive practices as outlined in this chapter. In addition, the anonymous nature of cyberspace creates uncertainty concerning who is actually participating. If the following two assumptions have merit, however, then the balance shifts away from who the participants are (e.g. their physical identities) and towards what they can bring to the table: (1) that ordinary people are more competent than anyone else to decide when and how much they shall intervene on decisions they feel are important to them (Dahl 1970: 35); and (2) that who somebody is remains less salient to identifying and articulating problems than what is revealed in their speech and action, for example the content of their messages (Arendt 1958: 179). Of course, it is critical that the content of cyberspace be diverse and that universal access to these forums continues to be a hallmark of US telecommunications policy. The strong correlation between socio-economic status and ownership rates of basic and advanced telecommunications services, including computers, belies this ideal. Even if diverse groups participate in political forums, social psychology research shows that homogeneity of in-group members tends to be an important feature of minority groups, new groups and groups with well-defined agendas, such as political groups. If norms can be established in which bridges are built connecting diverse political newsgroups, such as promoting intergroup dialogue, then at the very least the perception of in-group members towards out-groups might be changed. Another direction might be to normalise a right of reply. Perhap the design of the network, including facilitation and moderation, can enable citizens more effectively to respond to and incorporate others' viewpoints, so that collective action is as regular an occurrence online as, say, contacting the White House.

Appendix: universe of Usenet political newsgroups and AOL forums

Usenet political newsgroups

alt.politics.black.helicopters
alt.politics.british
alt.politics.bush
alt.politics.clinton
alt.politics.correct
alt.politics.corruption.mena
alt.politics.datahighway
alt.politics.democratics.d
alt.politics.ec
alt.politics.economics
x-alt.politics.elections
alt.politics.equality
alt.politics.europe.misc
alt.politics.greens
alt.politics.homosexuality
alt.politics.immigration
alt.politics.italy
alt.politics.korea
x-alt.politics.liberation
x-alt.politics.media
alt.politics.meijer
alt.politics.nationalism.black
alt.politics.nationalism.white
alt.politics.org.batf
x-alt.politics.org.cia
alt.politics.org.fbi
alt.politics.org.misc
alt.politics.org.nsa
alt.politics.org.un
alt.politics.perot
alt.politics.radical-left
x-alt.politics.reform
alt.suburbs
alt.politics.sex
alt.politics.socialism.mao
alt.politics.socialism.trotsky
alt.politics.usa.congress
alt.politics.usa.constitution
alt.politics.usa.misc
alt.politics.usa.newt-gingrich
alt.politics.usa.republican
alt.politics.vietnamese
x-alt.politics.white-power

alt.politics.youth
talk.politics.animals
talk.politics.china
talk.politics.crypto
talk.politics.drugs
talk.politics.european-union
talk.politics.guns
talk.politics.libertarian
talk.politics.medicine
talk.politics.mideast
talk.politics.misc
talk.politics.soviet
talk.politics.theory
talk.politics.tibet

AOL's 'Washington Connection'	
x-Abortion	Gun Control
x-Decision 96	Immigration
Domestic Issues	International Issues
Federal Budget and Taxes	Pending Legislation
The Fence Post	x-Political Viewpoint
Forum Feedback	x-Welfare
General Debate	White House

Note: 'x' indicates forums randomly chosen for content analysis

11 Deweyan systems in the Information Age

G. Scott Aikens

In free countries, there is often found more real public wisdom and sagacity in shops and manufactories than in the cabinets of princes in countries where no one dares to have an opinion until he comes into them.

Edmund Burke, in a 1780 address to his fellow British elites in defence of the American revolutionaries

Foreground

The Information Age is characterised by the growth of contradictory forces. Twenty-first century institutions will be forged by efforts to resolve these tensions. In this chapter, I focus on systems of decision making.

On the one hand, in *The Rise of the Network Society*, Manuel Castells portrays an increasingly powerful global elite, sharing information and using complex media strategies to influence democratic elections and public policy processes. Castells calls this 'media politics'. Important amongst the tools of media politics are the bodies of knowledge held by teams of producers, pollsters, marketers and consultants. The power of television is central to these experts in shaping public opinion. Castells refers to scandal politics – sensationalistic TV stories used as tools to sway emotions of the mass electorate to achieve political ends – as a crucial part of media politics. This cynical disregard by elites of public opinion is an increasingly dominant and worrying trend.

On the other hand, Castells proposes that new interactive technologies that transform control over the flow of information and ideas might be used to create new deliberative mechanisms. He cites early examples of how distributed networks serve to mobilise issue-based groups, such as environmentalists and the American militia movement. Castells concludes that,

> if political representation and decision-making could find a linkage with these new sources of input from concerned citizenry without yielding to a savvy technological elite, a new kind of civil society could be reconstructed, thus allowing for the electronic grassrooting of democracy.
>
> (Castells 1997: 352)

In line with this latter possibility, pioneering work aimed at using new technologies to create deliberative forums integrated formally into existing representative structures has been taking place for several years. Although the new technologies are very much a product of the American imagination, the path of development has, for this author, included both North America and Europe.[1] Let me briefly review some of this work.

In 1994, a group of us in Minnesota configured the first interactive political site on the internet, called Minnesota E-Democracy (http://e-democracy.org). That same year I organised two electronic debates (E-Debates) between candidates for the US Senate and Governor of Minnesota, thus formally wiring the net into the democratic process for the first time. These were gatewayed into MN-POLITICS, an e-mail forum with over 700 citizen-participants (Aikens 1998: 1–9). This simple e-mail network has become stronger over the years, hosting E-Debates each election cycle, styling itself as a champion of civic liberal ideals in the US. Not only do citizens, activists, journalists and public servants participate regularly in the network, but so did the main operatives for the leading contenders in the 1998 gubernatorial race. As David Thune said of MN-POLITICS when he was President of St Paul City Council:

> In terms of government and politics, it's like zero steps removed. It's a direct one-on-one communication, therefore democracy. It's as close to the one person, one vote concept as you can get. Every individual not only has a voice but also an ear on the other end to hear what they think.
>
> (Featherly)

This experience led to my involvement in British politics, where I've participated in two projects that use Minnesota as a model. The first of these, UK Citizens Online Democracy (see Chapter 1), supported by Prime Minister Blair, is a non-profit, non-partisan electronic network founded in 1996 for citizen politics in the mould of Minnesota (http://www.democracy.org.uk). It seeks to promote civic education and participatory democracy locally, nationally and, perhaps, on a European-wide scale. The 'OPEN' forum is a central hub for the site, modelled on MN-POLITICS (see Gallagher).

The second project, Nexus – the policy and ideas network, is the UK's first virtual think tank, intended to open out the policy process and develop the ideas that will shape the agendas of governments (http://www.nctnexus.org). As Tony Blair wrote in the context of Nexus at the time of its founding in 1996,

> There is a pressing need for continued debate to deepen these ideas, refine them, toughen them up. People outside the party have a critical role. They can help us understand the issues and forces shaping society so that we can shape the future.
>
> (Blair 1996)

From 1996 to 1998, Nexus hosted conferences, seminars and online consultations. During the early years, online events addressed issues such as higher education policy in the UK and the impact of information and communication technologies on society. In February 1998, Nexus was invited to use UK-POLICY, an e-mail forum modelled on MN-POLITICS, to run a consultation for the Prime Minister's Policy Unit about the nature of the 'third way' between old left and new right (Thompson and Aikens 1998: 22–3). This erupted into a passionate debate and was followed by a flurry of press reports and a seminar at 10 Downing Street. In the days succeeding the seminar, Prime Minister Blair submitted a message to UK-POLICY:

> The Nexus internet discussion of the Third Way has been a unique experiment in political debate. It has shown the potential of the new medium to be serious, constructive and imaginative, with interventions from around the world. I am happy to congratulate the organisers, and look forward to taking forward the ideas raised at the NEXUS seminar scheduled for Thursday 7th May.

This hints at the impact the online deliberation had, as does the summary paper, http://www.netnexus.org/3way:

Politics is changing and I believe the left-of-centre has the opportunity, and special responsibility, to develop the ideas that will shape the debates of the new century. Clear in our values, we must combine analytical insight into the way the world is changing, with genuine imagination about how to put our values into effect. The Nexus discussion of the Third Way has made an important contribution to that project and I look forward to further debates.

In this chapter, I wish to outline the intellectual framework for Minnesota E-Democracy and, to an extent therefore, UKCOD and Nexus. This account focuses on a debate between the journalist-philosopher Walter Lippmann and the philosopher and leading progressive John Dewey during the 1920s. Lippmann, a central progenitor of today's media politics, set out to formalise the role of media in American systems of decision making as radio and then television were becoming important. Dewey was a leader of the American progressive movement during the early part of the twentieth century and sought to think through a communications system to support a new politics of individual freedom within cohesive communities. I propose that the projects described above can be viewed fruitfully as Deweyan systems, intended to counter the dangerous tendencies of modern media politics.

Before proceeding, it is necessary to note that the exchanges between Dewey and Lippmann are a provincial American debate. As such, this treatment is most applicable to the American context. Of course, the American mass media is a powerful global phenomenon and, as the above demonstrates, the new American-made technologies are also a global phenomenon. This limited treatment is, therefore, a contribution to international dialogue. As I mention in conclusion, creating a strong framework for comparative research to navigate transformation ought to be a priority.

Walter Lippmann

Walter Lippmann, working on propaganda for the United States during the First World War, became concerned with the relations between decision-making systems and ways in which the new media influence public opinion. In his classic book of 1922, *Public Opinion*, Lippmann sets out a blueprint for how systems ought to develop, with a particular interest in links to the public. The book outlines a need and a plan to retool American democracy to meet modern conditions.

In light of the 'war to make the world safe for democracy', it became clear to Lippmann that too many in the US continue to adhere to democratic ideals in a world in which these are unrealisable. Thomas Jefferson expressed a near mystical faith in the ability of the people to govern themselves. As Lippmann writes, 'The democratic ideal, as Jefferson moulded it . . . became the political gospel, and supplied the stereotypes through which Americans of all parties have looked at politics' (Lippmann 1960: 270). This continues to this day, with Al Gore suggesting that the internet be built on a Jeffersonian architecture, and Newt Gingrich naming the congressional information locator Thomas, in honour of Jefferson. Yet, in Lippmann's view, the Jeffersonian vision was always and forever ill-suited to the needs of a vast, technologically advanced, commercial nation-state. It may be useful as a tool of communication between politicians and the public, but there was for Lippmann a structural need to move beyond a naïve faith in popular self-government.

According to Lippmann, democratic idealists naïvely assume that people are well enough informed to possess sound judgements on matters of state. Famously, he investigates the flaws in this proposition. To discharge a democratic function successfully a person would, realistically, have to have a phenomenal grasp of local, national and international affairs. This person would have to be 'omni-competent' when, in reality, people construct for themselves a conception of the world based on 'fictions', 'symbols', 'fragments' and 'stereotypes', or, as Lippmann titled the introductory chapter of his book, 'pictures in our heads'. He concludes, 'Not being omni-present and omni-scient we cannot see much of what we have to think and talk about' (ibid.: 161).

For Lippmann, this portrait of fragmentation is at odds with the needs of decision making in contemporary societies. He writes, 'How, in the language of democratic theory, do great numbers of people feeling each so privately about so abstract a picture develop any common will?'. In broaching the topic of the 'common will', Lippmann suggests that an 'Oversoul' is necessary. This Oversoul is the crystallisation of the nation-wide wishes of an informed and active citizen-body, acting in concert to create legislation and govern itself. In other words, it is the crystallisation of a fiction. Instead, the consent of the governed must be constructed by living human beings. He writes, 'the Oversoul as presiding genius in corporate behaviour is a superfluous mystery if we fix our attention upon the machine'. Lippmann thus follows his conclusion that democratic ideals are an impossibility with another conclusion: a minority will always dominate. He writes, 'Nowhere is the idyllic theory of democracy realised. . . . There is an inner circle, surrounded by concentric circles which fade out gradually into the disinterested or uninterested rank and file' (ibid.: 228).

To systematise a formal move from democratic naïveté to reality, Lippmann proposes the replacement of devotion to the democratic ideal of self-government with devotion to the achievement of a high standard of living as a gauge for the good society. By defining results on the basis of 'a standard of living in which man's capacities are properly exercised', the entire problem of political organisation changes. With the emphasis on producing 'a certain minimum of health, housing, material necessities, education, freedom, pleasure', etc., the 'criteria can be made exact and objective, which is inevitably the concern of comparatively few people' (ibid.: 314).

The driving force behind such a change is the deep allegiance on the part of key sectors of society to the ideal of success. In America, this ideal is most notably symbolised by a simple doctrine of mechanical progress which fosters a desire 'for the biggest, the fastest, the highest, or if you are a maker of wrist-watches or microscopes, the smallest; the love, in short, of the superlative and the peerless'. Conveniently, the key sectors, including Lippmann, that promote the young American meritocracy are those deemed by their standards of living the best. These are the 'comparatively few' who control the machinery of governance.

Lippmann argues that elite policy-making bodies and privately owned media systems will perpetuate this realistic new status quo. This would be done by expert intelligence in government and by raising the achievement of a high standard of living to a public ideal – the American Dream. Political power resides in the machinery propounding the new ideal. Lippmann writes, 'the pattern has been a success so nearly perfect in the sequence of ideals, practice, and results, that any challenge to it is called un-American' (ibid.: 110).

Three inter-related elements central to the systems of decision making proposed by Lippmann are: the construction of a system of 'organised intelligence' in elite administrative circles; the subsumption of political communication under the economics of mass media; and the creation of a culture of 'objectivity' in the journalistic profession.

First, for Lippmann, the key to strong systems of governance is the creation of 'organised intelligence' in the form of centrally located intelligence agencies, staffed by professional scientists, social scientists and administrators. The pivotal nexus of power is vested in these highly rational policy elites, which have invested the time and energy in understanding the complex functioning of the modern nation-state. Lippmann writes, 'Only by insisting that problems shall not come up to him until they have passed through a procedure, can the busy citizen of a modern state hope to deal with these in a form that is intelligible.' (ibid.: 402).

Second, the political media must function as a subsidiary sphere of the mass media. The point of the mass media is to run a profitable business by reaching the largest audience possible. For an idealistic democrat, this creates a tension between the general motive of profit maximisation and the special role of the political media in informing public opinion on affairs of the state. As Lippmann puts it, 'We expect the newspaper to serve us with truth however unprofitable the truth may be'. The fact that the media organisation makes the most money by selling advertising space forces the editor to be cognisant of the interests and opinions of current and potential advertisers (the successful). By subjecting the construction of political media to these pressures, Lippmann portrays a certain kind of system of accountability. The decision-making abilities of the news editor, acting as intermediary between the public and government, are constrained by the weight of opinion of the business community that funds the product.

Finally, Lippmann formulates the importance of objectivity within the news process. To Lippmann's mind, a happening becomes news when it can be 'fixed, objectified, measured, named'. A dispute, for example, becomes news when there is an arrest, or a complaint filed in a court. A 'dangerous issue' such as a strike – to take Lippmann's example – becomes news only when there is a concrete record of an action in some institution or when there is an event that disturbs the day-to-day activity of the citizen. Thus, in the case of the strike, the news is 'the indisputable fact and the easy interest ... the strike itself and the readers' inconvenience'. One of several reasons offered for standards of objectivity is the desire of the editor to have a professional operation and rules of the game. The staff will thus have guidelines to help them avoid offending, confusing or alienating the loyal reader and/or advertiser with unconventional, insufficient or clumsily described material.

John Dewey

In the 1920s, philosopher John Dewey expressed a great deal of admiration for Lippmann's work, writing that it is no longer possible to look at democracy in the same way after absorbing *Public*

Opinion.[2] In his assimilation of the analysis, however, Dewey opens out problematic territory.

Dewey admits that Lippmann is right: a congress of autonomous local communities was the basis upon which the democratic ideal of self-government was supposed to function, according to traditional democrats. Circumstances have made such an environment an anachronism. Time and events render the democratic ideal of self-government impractical and unworkable in the vast, complex nation-state that has developed.

Dewey also agrees that this is caught up in the complexity of the Machine Age. Driven by steam, cable, telephone, radio, the railway, cheap printing and mass production, the Machine Age is deeply marked by what President Woodrow Wilson termed the 'new era of human relations'. Men and women are closely linked by distant events through the rapid communication of information and transportation of material goods. A primary consequence of the Machine Age and the new era of human relations is the significance of events beyond their grasp to individuals living in local communities scattered across a vast nation-state. This extreme reliance of local people on the business of the nation is responsible for the fragmentation of and deterioration in the significance of the local community in the day-to-day life of the individual. As Dewey puts it, 'the machine age in developing the Great Society has invaded and partially disintegrated the small communities of former times' (Dewey 1927: 127).

Finally, Dewey agrees with Lippmann about the importance of the machinery by which consent to govern is forged, such as systems of expertise and press. Dewey understands that communication systems are essential to the organisation of power, writing that 'The smoothest road to control over political conduct is by control of opinion' (ibid.: 182).

Dewey does not, however, agree with Lippmann's plan to eliminate the principle of democratic self-government in favour of the American Dream of Success and to create systems of decision making that perpetuate the new Ideal as a gauge for the good society. Such plans for decision-making systems that compartmentalise expertise and centralise control of ideas may work in current conditions, especially given tendencies towards complexity, but they are too crude. They prioritise the need to concentrate power to govern over the need to think about the power of the individual to govern his or her personal domain. Dewey writes, 'Whatever obstructs and restricts publicity, limits and distorts public opinion and checks and distorts thinking on social affairs' (ibid.: 177).

With organised intelligence, decisions will be controlled by a tight caste of meritocratic elites protected from the increasingly fragmented thinking of a vast public. No matter how talented the lucky few, they are a population biased by success. No matter how well intentioned, they cannot adequately understand the needs of those for whom they make decisions. This compartmentalisation will result in an absence of common knowledge in the thinking of those guiding policy, laying the fate of political communities in the hands of a select few, which can only exacerbate inequality, as these few will be inclined to follow their own self-interest.

Additionally, the privatisation of cumbersome communication systems will mean that the flow of ideas is tightly constrained by the interests of financiers. Furthermore, there will be few safeguards against the possibility that competition will cause an increasing rate of centralisation, leading to systems increasingly controlled by even more powerful financiers. Such centralisation of power over ideas throughout the political community does not truly reflect the complexity of human interconnectedness. In proposing systems that dismiss self-government, Lippmann dismisses the importance of individual identity within the political community. Without adequate vehicles for civic participation, it will be difficult to build a robust enough sense of political agency for the individual to fulfil the rights and responsibilities of citizenship in a free society. This will result in an impoverished conception of citizenship.

The 'American Dream of life, liberty and the pursuit of happiness' will be rotted by the 'American Dream of Success', as the capacity of individuals to manage their affairs is undermined to make management easier for the select few. If the tradition of personal liberty with the logic of distribution built into the system design has a basis that is more sound than the corporatist philosophy of success, such an assault will have negative macroscopic consequences. For example, an impoverished sense of citizenship in a significant segment of the population will result in a decline in normative standards of behaviour in all areas of life, patterns of irresponsibility and ongoing erosion of the social fabric through neglect. This will show itself statistically in deteriorating standards in families, institutions and communities. On-going maintenance of frayed institutions will become a drain on economic and psychic energies, depleting the resources necessary for sustained social and economic well-being, making a mockery of the ideal of success itself.

Dewey argued that the decision-making systems promoted by Lippmann would not last. Robust participation in decision-making systems is necessary to serve a variety of functions for the well-being of social fabric and economic life. Dewey believed that advances in science would produce communication systems sophisticated enough to address the difficulties he perceived in the work of Lippmann. Thus, where Lippmann argued that neither the press nor any other institution compensates for 'the failure of self-governing people to transcend their casual experience and their prejudices by inventing, creating and organising a machinery of knowledge', Dewey wrote, 'When the machine age has thus perfected its machinery it will be a means of life and not its despotic master. Democracy will come into its own, for democracy is a name for a life of free and enriching communication'.

During the 1920s, however, Dewey feared that the set of developments summarised as both the Machine Age and the era of new human relations favoured the ideals promoted by Lippmann. On the positive side, he asserted that the literature of democracy, with ideals on self-government, 'retain their glamour and sentimental prestige' and 'still engage thought and command loyalty'. On the negative side, given the patterns of development in telegraphy and radio, he concluded, 'those which have actual instrumentalities at their disposal have the advantage' (ibid.: 184).

From then to now

Research is accumulating that supports Dewey's hypothesis about the importance of interconnectedness as well as the reality of decline. For example, Robert Putnam (1993b) proposes that we call this basic civic interaction 'social capital'. Like Dewey, he proposes that a high incidence of robust interaction or social capital within the community throughout the course of daily life is essential to the working of a healthy democracy. Putnam (1996) has charted the declining rates of civic participation beginning after the depressions-era generation, and has suggested that this is indicative of declining social capital, which is a worrying trend. Others, including Putnam, are beginning to pull together evidence on why this is worrying, by demonstrating the importance of social capital to long-term economic well-being, particularly in an increasingly networked society (see Halpem 1998 and Szreter).

Putnam comes even closer to a Deweyan analysis about the adverse effects of Lippmanesque systems when he proposes television as a primary cause of the erosion of social capital. Whilst Putnam does not specifically focus on social capital and political communication, there does seem to be a strong correlation between the Deweyan critique of Lippmann and the worrying acceleration of media politics and scandal politics described by Castells. Over time, the abandonment of distributed system design in favour of compartmentalisation and centralisation spurred by competition, erodes measures that might prevent political operatives and media professionals from using increasingly corrupt methods that undermine the system (see Grossman 1995 and Fallow 1996). At the same time, people's awareness of being raised into political structures that do not enable them to perform the functions of citizenship adequately may become manifest in distrust of those structures. In this way, deteriorating social capital may cause decline in political trust. If social capital and political trust are key to long-term economic well-being in a networked society, understanding these trends and creating counter-measures could become a priority for nations

The roots of the internet mesh well with Deweyan thinking about the role of scientific investigation as a model for democratic practice, supporting a belief that humanity has an aptitude for self-correction in system design. During the Second World War, Vannevar Bush, as Director of the American Office of Scientific Research, was responsible for the work done by physicists on behalf of the war effort. After the war and under the weight of the emerging nuclear threat, Bush attempted to inspire the community of physicists to apply their skills to perfecting a new machinery of knowledge. In *The Atlantic Monthly* in 1945, Bush wrote:

> The application of science have built man a well-supplied house, and are teaching him to live healthily therein. They have enabled him to throw masses of people against another with cruel weapons. They may yet allow him truly to encompass the great record and to grow in the wisdom of race experience. He may perish in conflict before he learns to wield that record for his true good. Yet, in the application of science to the needs and desires of man, it would seem to be a singularly unfortunate stage at which to terminate the process, or to lose hope as to the outcome.
>
> (Bush 1945)

Bush's vision was carried through the 1960s and 1970s by the 'geeks' working on the ARPANET project. United by their scientific intelligence and independent spirits, these men knew that if a Soviet missile took one node out of the network, others would maintain communication and the spirit of independence would survive. It wasn't socialism: it was a social way to preserve personal liberty. Furthermore, Fernando Corbato and Robert Fano of MIT, who developed key concepts such as time sharing, envisioned how distributed systems would enable this new machinery of knowledge to work for the benefit of community collaboration. They wrote:

> The time-sharing computer system can unite a group of investigators in a co-operative search for the solution to a common problem, or it can serve as a community pool of knowledge and skill on which anyone can draw according to his needs. Projecting the concept on a large scale, one can conceive of such a facility as an extraordinarily powerful library serving an entire community, a sort of intellectual public utility.
>
> (Corbato and Fano 1966: 76)

Today the logic of distributed systems dominates the market and seems to transform everything, including the crude systems of yesterday. The availability and speed of new technologies has changed and will continue to change the way in which people interact with one another, and how ideas flow locally, regionally and globally. The newest generation of technology provides the end-user with communication tools that are relatively cheaper yet significantly more powerful than anything previously available. In reconfiguring the ways in which humans interact, the economic and technological factors shaping developments transform the control of information and knowledge. Substantial change in the political economy of information distribution and human communication will go hand in hand with change in the very constitution of society.

Deweyan systems in the Information Age

Lippmann and Dewey agreed that political power lies in communication machinery configured to perpetuate ideals. In the light of the proposed importance of social capital and political trust to long-term economic well-being, a machinery of knowledge may be needed to perpetuate Deweyan ideals. It may be necessary to bring civic interaction and self-government back into the gauge for a good society. With distributed systems as the building blocks of a new machinery of knowledge, a new politics of personal liberty within socially cohesive communities might be a realistic aim.

I have taken some preliminary steps in trying to realise this plan and have gained confidence in its viability through experience. Quite simply, I have placed e-mail forums at points where the logic of distributed systems creates new publics in which decision makers can take part or observe. The key is to craft rules of civic engagement that arise out of the logic by doing the minimum required to sustain civic spaces.

In open online forums such as MN-POLITICS, OPEN and UK-POLICY, for example, participants have the opportunity to contribute but also the responsibility for what they do. They can say anything, but if it's silly or aggressive or offensive, others can react, or ignore. This makes people think about what they're doing, and maybe about who they are. Of course, sometimes people don't think and continue with behaviour that jeopardises the well-being of the forum. The guidelines for civic engagement used by all the forums are successful because they do the minimum necessary to preserve freedom of participation. People are forced to think about the community, as each individual is equally responsible for the group's survival. It won't last if participants don't control what they say, and it will if they do.

Furthermore, as perspectives accumulate, including those of people who have lived through and shaped the history in question, the complexity of context becomes uniquely tangible. The combination of a tangible context and the on-going freedom of the forum bounded by rules of civic engagement is a powerful combination, leading to intensive exploration of context. This is a system of decision making far more sophisticated than traditional media politics, in which economic bottlenecks to communication cause the fetishisation of the vote, forcing debate to be constrained in advance for the sake of being 'on-message'. With the new medium, it becomes possible for ideas to be challenged, dismissed, accepted, refined and/or transformed into honed knowledge, creating the opportunity for a community logic to emerge, built on but separated from any given voice with its limited perspective.

These systems are neither utopian nor depressingly elitist. Rather, forums with guidelines can be models for the rights and responsibilities of personal liberty within socially cohesive communities. Perhaps these can catalyse transformation of existing systems, creating networks able to support a politics capable of reversing the worrying decline in social capital and political trust. Implementing the sophisticated technology for the task of self-correction is the aim.

If these systems are going to be powerful enough to deal with perceived macroscopic problems, however, development needs to go

much further. There is a need to think strategically about trans-
forming the flow of ideas nationally, locally and globally to buttress
the capacity for civic participation and self-government. An important element of this is to design systems that will alter patterns of
elite formation from compartmentalised and centralised systems to
distributed systems.[3]

Briefly, I will outline two general methods for navigating this
transformation towards democratic outcomes. First, learning from
the model of 'Nexus – the policy and ideas network', organised
intelligence can fruitfully be supplemented by multiple gateways to
socialised intelligence, so community logics will regularly infuse the
thinking of policy elites. Whilst Deweyan systems accept the need
for rich systems of organised intelligence in complex societies, these
can become richer through the active engagement of experts in open
and free decision-making systems at the local, regional and global
level. Knowledge separate from distribution amidst an open public
is not socialised knowledge. Dewey writes, 'No government by
experts in which the masses do not have the chance to inform the
experts as to their needs can be anything but an oligarchy managed
in the interests of the few.' Furthermore, it is not necessary that all
participants possess expertise, but it would create an important check
on power if all citizens possess the opportunity to judge the posted
positions of those who do possess expertise. Dewey writes,

> It is not necessary that the many should have the knowledge
> and skill to carry on the needed investigations: what is required
> is that they have the ability to judge the bearing of the knowl-
> edge supplied by others upon common concerns.
>
> (Dewey 1927: 209)

Second, the need to integrate decision-making systems into local
communities is obviously one of the most important requirements
for the creation of social capital, political trust and as an aid to
long-term economic well-being. Learning from the Minnesota E-
Democracy model, Deweyan systems are, therefore, rooted in local
community. Dewey writes, 'Only when we start from a community
as a fact, grasp the fact in thought so as to clarify and enhance its
constituent elements, can we reach an idea of democracy which is
not Utopian' (ibid.: 149).

Local systems can serve a number of functions, of which I will
mention two. First, robust communities result from a robust conception of citizenship that emphasises civic education and active

participation. Deweyan systems can act as lifelong training programmes in self-government by creating vehicles for both training and regular practice in governing one's self in one's political community. The key is to teach an individual how to be a citizen rather than expect individuals to control the destiny of a state by referendum.

Second, when formally integrated into the political process, these systems can become new institutions of accountability on an ongoing basis. As Dewey writes, 'Only through constant watchfulness and criticism of public officials by citizens can a state be maintained in integrity and usefulness' (ibid.: 69). Where, for Lippmann, a suspect notion of journalistic objectivity is a primary system of accountability, distributed systems allow for community logics beyond the compass of single perspectives to emerge, and these are powerful engines of accountability.

Conclusion

A theoretical foundation is being developed to guide activity, and new institutions are emerging. Experiences in the field demonstrate the viability of the foundation and provide data for refinement. There is, however, a long way to go before Deweyan systems are the norm.

The conscious organisation by policy and industrial leaders of processes for navigating new systems of decision making in a global information society is needed. I believe that this exists in embryo through the interplay of research and practice hinted at above. Knowledge gained through experience in the field can guide the continuing development of international research, with mechanisms for refined knowledge being circulated amongst decision makers and practitioners, flowing back to designers to develop new processes. I believe the groundwork has been prepared. The crucial step is for leaders to become conscious of the project.

Notes

1 My work results from my American imagination and a European education. Cambridge academics such as John Dunn and Quentin Skinner have been influential. For example, as Dunn writes 'What modern politics most pressingly requires is a democratisation of prudence, a spreading out of the burden of judging and choosing soberly about political questions across the entire adult populations of specific societies' (Dunn, 1990).
2 For more information on Dewey see, e.g., Westerbrook, (1991) and (1995).

3   This may already be happening in the US in a haphazard fashion. For example, the economist Robert J. Samuelson says that new technologies threaten the income, social importance and political influence of the 'media elite' who run the TV networks and large newspapers. This view is supported by a survey from the Pew Research Centre for the People and the Press, showing a shift in the audience for TV networks' nightly news programmes. In 1993, these were regularly watched by 60% of Americans over 18, compared to 38% in 1998. At the same time, in 1995 4% of adults used the internet to get news once a week, compared to 20% today (*The Washington Post*, July 8 1998, pg. A17; http://www.washingtonpost.com/wp-srv/WPlate/1998–07/08/0201–070898 -idx.html.

12 Cutting out the middle man: from virtual representation to direct deliberation

Stephen Coleman

The multitude, for the moment, is foolish, when they act without deliberation.

Introduction

In 1796, when Edmund Burke wrote the above words, less than one in twenty of the British population had the vote. Qualified by nothing more than the ownership of property, this minority perceived itself to be justified in representing the interests of the less affluent, less educated majority. Such justification for electoral oligarchy was referred to as *virtual representation*. It rested upon the assumption of political trusteeship: the notion of 'an aristocracy of virtue and wisdom governing for the good of the whole nation' (Pitkin 1967: 172). Burke estimated that no more than 400,000 people possessed sufficient leisure time for discussion, access to the means of information and sufficient wealth to place them above menial dependence. 'This is the British publick', declared Burke, meaning that this minority was entitled to representative status in virtue of the general public. The claimed necessity for representative trusteeship was itself predicated upon the alleged incapacity of the mass of the public to reason for themselves. Burke conceded that 'the most poor, illiterate and uninformed creatures upon earth are judges of *practical* oppression' but this does not enable them to understand the cause of or remedy for their problems. From discussion of such matters they

> ought to be totally shut out; because their reason is weak; because when once aroused, their passions are ungoverned; because they want information; because the smallness of the property, which they individually possess, renders them less attentive to the measures they adopt in affairs of moment.
>
> (Burke 1846–8)

Lord North, speaking in opposition to a failed motion for electoral reform, posed himself a rhetorical question which he proceeded to answer in accordance with the prevailing orthodoxy of virtual representation: 'Did freedom depend upon every individual subject being represented in that House? Certainly not; for that House, constituted as it was, represented the whole Kingdom' (Dickinson 1977: 286). So, according to this fundamentally elitist theory of representation, the disenfranchised poor could rest contented that they were voted for by the enfranchised rich. Manchester, represented directly by no seat in parliament, was nonetheless virtually represented by the city of Bristol; and the electors of Bristol, whose MP was Edmund Burke, should not mistake representation for delegation, for, as Burke unashamedly told them, 'Parliament is a deliberative assembly' and deliberation was the prerogative of representatives rather than voters.

Although there has clearly been a progression from virtual representation, with voting confined to a minority of the population (4.1 per cent in 1831, 16.4 per cent in 1868, 30 per cent in 1914), to actual representation via universal franchise (74 per cent by 1921), the Burkean dichotomy between voting and deliberating has persisted into contemporary politics. With the rise of the broadcast media, a style of politics evolved that emphasised the role of voters as spectators upon the deliberations of the Great and the Good. From the Oxbridge Senior Common Room flavour of debate from above, epitomised by the BBC's highly successful *Brains Trust* programmes of the 1940s, to the grudging acceptance of cameras in parliament in the late 1980s, an implicit ethos of *virtual deliberation* has emerged. Citizens watch and listen to the elite thinking aloud on behalf of the public. The agenda of discussion tends to be set by party communication managers (the infamous spin doctors) and senior media editors, both locked into a systemic process of mutual dependence and ultimate monopoly over the production both of news and publicly mediated discussion. This manifestation of public politics as a form of public relations was described by Habermas as undermining the condition within which an open public sphere of rational critical discussion may take place; in its place had emerged a 'refeudalisation of the public sphere', leaving citizens rather like peasant onlookers at the affairs of the Royal Court (Habermas 1989). Blumler and Gurevitch, after many years of analysing the way in which political communication takes place, especially within the context of empirical accounts of media-dominated election campaigns, concluded that an 'impoverishing way of addressing citizens about political issues has been gaining an institutionally rooted hold that seems inherently difficult to resist or shake off' (Blumler and Gurevitch 1996: 203). The resultant 'crisis of political communication', as the latter writers have referred to it, is less an academic postulation than an observable civic disengagement from the political process 'as seen on TV'. According to the ITC Report on public views of broadcasting during the 1997 UK general election, voters are distinctly uninterested in TV elections: although 74 per cent of those polled by the ITC said that election coverage was important, only 37 per cent said that they were interested in watching it; 41 per cent of 16–24 year olds said that they switched channels or switched off rather than watch election coverage. Millions actually did switch off from election news programmes, which actually suffered a decline in ratings during the key election campaign period: 60 per cent of those surveyed said that there was too much election news; audience ratings for the BBC *Nine O'Clock News* fell by a fifth, and yet as many as 25 per cent of the electorate were undecided about how to vote when the campaign started. (Could this have been the same quarter of the population – the highest proportion since 1935 – who in 1997 simply did not bother to vote?) Such cynicism and apathy exists within the broader context of a general public belief in the impotence and futility of political participation (Rowntree 1996).

Interactive discourse

There is a form of technological determinism that regards essentially monological media, such as radio and TV, as inimical to public participation, whilst new media, such as the internet, possess inherently dialogical, democratic and libertarian characteristics, allowing political communication to return to the people. The latter, sanguine assumption may be true, insofar as many-to-many communication networks are structurally unsuited to centralised agenda or content control. Even so, there is no automatically democratic character to the new media; democratic practice must be established within political culture, not depended upon as if it were an inevitable property of a technological package. Similarly, it is a mistake to regard the virtual deliberation of broadcasting as a technologically inherent feature. In fact, many of the arguments for the free communication conditions often claimed for the internet could have been applied to the potentialities within early radio production (which need not have developed corporately, but for the politico-economic culture within which it was born) and were indeed applied by many optimistic commentators in the early days of cable TV (Engelman 1990).

The element of interactive discourse, which is often presented as the inherently democratic factor within the communicative structure of new media technologies, had emerged within the womb of the old media. The combination of radio studio and simple telephone technology produced the new format of the phone-in programme, which began in Britain in the late 1960s – some time after it had taken root in the USA. Phone-in interactivity profoundly affected the hitherto vocal passivity of broadcast audiences. Indeed, at this point in history, the interactive experience of questioning a politician on a nationally broadcast phone-in programme is likely to be much more politically satisfying and objectively influential than expressing and exchanging opinions about politics in an online news group. One need only contrast the BBC *Election Call* series, broadcast in every UK election since 1974 and now simulcast on TV and radio, with the April 1998 Prime Ministerial webcast. In the former broadcasts, citizens could phone directly and inexpensively to put questions or points of view to politicians, including the party leaders. The process was mediated in a number of ways that have been the subject of extensive research by the present writer; but, however controlled the occasion, there was a transparent spontaneity about the interaction between callers (including highly critical citizens) and those competing to represent them. Fifty-nine per cent of viewers/listeners surveyed concluded that the programmes helped members of the public to play their part in setting the election agenda; 53 per cent said that callers were raising questions that they would have wanted to ask; and 64 per cent reported that *Election Call* provided an authentic voice for the public (Coleman *et al* 1999. The Prime Ministerial webcast, by contrast, was limited not only to the usual minority of citizens with internet access, but to those possessing special proprietorial software (produced by Microsoft); bandwidth limitations meant that no more than 5,000 people could listen to the webcast in real time; and those wanting to ask questions to the Prime Minister had to submit them four days in advance, apparently for unexplained technical reasons, but certainly to the political advantage of the webcast producers based at Number Ten.

Another contrast, in Northern Ireland, where there is a distinct vitality and significance to inclusive political communication, is between online discussion, which tends to involve a small minority of the population, often segregated virtually as in real life along

Cutting out the middle person 199

sectarian lines, and *Talkback*, BBC Radio Ulster's daily phone-in programme. In moments of high political tension, the latter programme
has provided a unique public sphere in which people who would never
normally exchange views are free to do so. During one week, as the
sectarian showdown in Drumcree unfolded, one in fifty of the
Northern Irish population aged over 16 called to put their views on
Talkback (Coleman 1998). Nothing approaching such a level of active
participation or public influence has yet been witnessed as a result of
online discussion in Northern Irish news groups.

The way in which citizens in society deliberate is as significant
for a functioning democracy as the way in which they cast votes.
The question of communicative presentation of ideas is no less
important than constitutional representation. So, just as actual representation in legislatures is a necessary but not sufficient condition
of democracy, actual rather than virtual deliberation within social
structures of communication is a democratic condition that must
also be achieved.

'[N]ew technology affords the possibility of cutting out ... (the)
middle person and directly inputting our views into the national,
regional and local electronic parliaments.' In these words, published
in *Wired* magazine, Graham Allen MP looked towards a new era
of direct deliberation. This is to be distinguished from direct democracy, in the sense of push-button plebiscites, as advocated by other
enthusiasts for the democratising powers of ICTs. Allen, the quin-
tessential constitutional moderniser, who has argued for the redesign
of the Westminster Parliament so as to make it less adversarial and
more electronically efficient, was advocating a form of interactive
relationship between parliamentary representatives and the represented via new channels of public information and deliberation. The
planners of the Scottish Parliament and Welsh assembly have assumed
the necessity of such interactive channels as a condition of a modern
democracy. The European Union's 1996 Green Paper, *Living and
Working in the Information Society: People First*, was no less optimistic about the capacity of new technologies to transform the nature
of representation: 'For true, inclusive democracy to exist, the whole
population must have equal access to information to make choices
effectively and equitably.... The vitality of political debate could
be reinvigorated through more use of direct democracy' (EU 1996:
101–2).

Indeed, the Westminster parliament, despite much talk of
modernising its procedures, has been slow to introduce the slightest
change in response to the new technologies. A 1998 consultation

by the Select Committee on the Modernisation of the House of Commons allowed MPs to consider modest proposals for secure electronic voting within the confines of the traditional Division Lobbies, but an overwhelming majority of MPs responded negatively on all counts. The Parliamentary Office of Science and Technology's Report on *Electronic Government*, which was innovative in scope whilst sober in tone, has been met with a conspicuous silence, even by the modernisers within Westminster (Coleman *et al* 1999).

The probable reason for the disinclination of many parliamentarians to trust new technologies, both in their own proceedings and as a means of enhancing their relationship with those whom they were elected to represent, is partly a result of being baffled by computers and partly an elitist sense that they hear quite enough from their constituents by post without opening up new channels of communication. Probably more influential than either of these reasons is a generally implicit belief that a more democratic culture of public communication would become inevitably subversive of representative government. The enthusiasts for direct democracy have tended to appropriate the discourse of ICTs as a political force (Becker 1981). In so doing, they have probably served to undermine the case for ICTs as a means of strengthening the democratic basis of representation. Techno-populism, as advocated by Ross Perot, Newt Gingrich and others in search of quick-fix appeals to 'the people's voice', has tended to regard the electronic *agora* as something akin to a vast opinion-polling exercise, or an ongoing national day-time talk show, neither of which bear much relationship to a model of direct deliberation in which informed citizens come to public judgement without being steered to moral consensus by Larry King or Jerry Springer. Government by gabfest will not enhance democracy.

Interactive communication technologies, including digital TV, with its immense capacity for return-path viewer-feedback, do possess the potential capacity to facilitate direct deliberation in ways that can connect citizens to the hitherto remote institutions of parliamentary representation. The question, therefore, is not whether such technologies can make democratic governance more accountable, but what kind of political channels need to be created to enable ICTs to become sources of public empowerment. Implementation of the following political mechanisms would go some way towards the realisation of direct public deliberation.

'Virtual public space'

The creation of a 'virtual public space' to enable citizens to inform themselves about issues of the day, scrutinise the workings of parliament and government, and enter into dialogue with decision makers in ways currently available to elites (often via expensive lobbying and shady cronyism) but rarely to average citizens.

Online policy proposals

A constitutional requirement for all local councils, national parliaments and assemblies and government departments to publish policy proposals online. How many citizens know about, let alone read and scrutinise, Green Papers, White Papers, EU Directives, local authority Development Plans or Bills being put before parliament? Just as *Hansard*, the daily record of parliamentary proceedings, is now available online, all proposed legislation should be accessible in the same way, not just so that citizens can inform themselves, but so that decision makers can be informed by citizens.

Online consultation

Regular pre-legislative online consultations, from the White Paper to the draft Bill stage, and again, perhaps, during the Standing Committee stage, in which the public will have its own 'virtual chamber' to deliberate on both the principles and details of major legislation. In 1997, the UK Cabinet Office supported an online public consultation to consider the White Paper proposal for a Freedom of Information Bill. This was the first such online consultation to be run in any nation-state.

Public involvement in Select Committees

Direct submission by citizens to Select Committees. Departmental Select Committees, established in 1979 as one of the most radical procedural innovations in parliamentary scrutiny, take regular submissions from expert witnesses. Proceedings could be webcast, with regular opportunities for members of the public to feed into inquiries, both as invited guests (via closed discussion lists) and within an open forum, accounts of which could be summarised and published as appendices to Select Committee reports.

Online conferences

The running of regular online conferences, hosted by Parliament, enabling wider groups of citizens to participate in policy deliberation, over a longer period of time than is afforded by one-day or half-day face-to-face meetings inside Parliament. Most meetings involving members of the public held in Parliament at the moment are limited, by necessity, to a narrow band of participants: those who are free during the day; those who can travel to London; those who are invited by MPs or other officials. Meetings are frequently rushed, with a Minister or MP delivering an opening address, documents of various lengths distributed and a pre-set agenda that has to be completed with a minimum of spontaneous revision. The result is that discussions are all too often compressed, over-controlled and limited to the Great and the Good. An online conference can include people from different parts of the country (or the world), without London being over-represented; it can allow participants more time to read online information, both before and during discussion; it can allow the agenda to be more flexible and determined by participants in response to their interacting interests; and it is archived for future reference, in contrast to the ephemerality of most face-to-face discussion meetings. Of course, an advantage of the latter is that participants have a chance to chat informally (during a tea break, over lunch or in a bar afterwards), whereas the offline potential for informal communication in online conferences may be less socially valuable. So, it is not a question of one type of meeting or the other; but at the moment most citizens never participate in any parliamentary or local authority meetings, and see the institution as remote, closed off and having nothing to do with them. Reports of online conferences can be produced and distributed to MPs and relevant officials.

Interactive information

The provision of regularly updated, interactive information about Parliament, including deliberative fora for citizens to exchange views with one another. The existing Parliament web site is distinctly non-interactive. Users could reasonably conclude from visiting http://www.parliament.uk that citizens' relationship with Parliament is expected to be purely passive. A 'people's forum' – or a series of fora on various policy issues – would have no political impact beyond the deliberative function of permitting people to talk with one another. Exchanging ideas in a free and open forum, without any votes being cast or politicians being lobbied, is itself a democratic act. Such fora could be used by school and college students as part of their studies in citizenship. Political literacy is best practised rather than simply taught.

Online evaluation

Online deliberative evaluations of policy areas could be established, involving random samples of the population. These could have an ongoing monitoring role, looking at such broad policy areas as welfare, constitutional change or Europe. They would be rather like standing focus groups, transparently evaluating and discussing policy, accountable not to parties, image makers or government institutions, but to their fellow citizens. Perhaps such standing deliberative lists could be organised regionally, to ensure diversity of deliberation. Online participants would control their own agendas, acting rather like Select Committees in choosing aspects of their particular policy areas to investigate and discuss.

None of the above proposals – some of which have been tried experimentally – is designed to replace representative democracy or to alter radically constitutionally established procedures of law making, parliamentary debate or scrutiny of the executive. The objective is to narrow the gap between representative administration and the deliberative input of the represented within a culture of democratic governance. In short, it is more a contribution to political culture than institutional government.

UKCOD

This is Britain's first national online democracy information and discussion service. It is an experiment which will evolve over the coming months to find out whether people can use online electronic communication to become better informed about and discuss the complex issues that affect their lives. We hope it will become a place to make things happen – a powerful new interface between the public and politicians, both locally and in the Palace of Westminster.

(UKCOD: 1996)

When UK Citizens Online Democracy (UKCOD) went online, with the above words as its opening declaration to the world, it was a severely underfunded organisation run by volunteers seeking to experiment with the possibility of creating a neutral public site in cyberspace where citizens could interact freely with one another and with those elected to represent them. The diverse group of citizens who set up UKCOD in 1995 were influenced by the experiences of various online democracy initiatives around the world, including the Minnesota E-Democracy project: a well-tested virtual forum that enabled the citizens of Minnesota to participate more deliberatively than ever before in the politics of their state. UKCOD began by experimenting with a number of online forums:

- a 1997 election discussion, focusing on two frequently marginalised policy areas (transport and constitutional reform);
- a first-time voters' forum in which the five main party leaders shared a 'virtual platform';
- an invitation-only debate on EMU, involving key EU figures;
- an online consultation about the last Conservative administration's *government.direct* Green Paper;
- a public consultation with the citizens of Brent, in which they were invited to propose the level of their council tax on the basis of information provided online;
- support for the Newham Youth Parliament, an initiative mainly run by young people from the east London borough;
- and collaboration with UK Communities Online, set up to encourage the online connectivity of every community in the UK.

By mid-1997, UKCOD had attained a level of public credibility to enable it to pioneer the UK's first ever pre-legislative online consultation. The Cabinet Office supported, but had no political control over, the *Have Your Say* web site, on which was published the Government's Freedom of Information White Paper; background information (including details of FOI laws in other countries, all *Hansard* references to FOI and newspaper articles on the subject); a chance for citizens to submit their comments on the White Paper to the Cabinet Office directly via the site; and a chance for citizens to put questions to the Minister in charge of the White Paper (David Clark) and judge his answers for themselves. The design of the site was tested, before it was launched publicly, on the people of Trimdon, County Durham, who had for some time been involved in a research project examining the effects of telematics on their post-industrial community. The people of Trimdon were unreserved in their criticism of the original site design, and within a short time it was redesigned along lines suggested by them and launched (Coleman and Loader forthcoming). In the first month after its launch, the majority of submissions in response to the White Paper came online from individual citizens; by the end of the consultation, only a third of all submissions came from individuals, with most coming from organised interest groups in paper form. Nonetheless, citizens who would previously never have put their views directly to the Cabinet Office were enabled to do so, and online submissions outnumbered those received on paper. The Prime Minister, Tony Blair, after being shown the site (by a group of schoolchildren), observed that

> The *Have Your Say* website is a historic opportunity for the public to play a meaningful part in the framing of new legislation. . . . I support this initiative to help modernise and enhance British democracy and open up Government and I hope similar consultations will be set up in future as part of the legislative process.

UKCOD had created a constitutional innovation which, if Blair's hope is realised, will serve as a precedent for the future of democratic governance.

Was the government influenced by the submissions on the UKCOD website? Were criticisms of the proposed legislation heeded in subsequent stages of the legislative process? Have users of the site become better informed as a result of it being there? Will the government have the courage to support similar consultations on issues more controversial than freedom of information? It is too early for these questions to be answered definitively. UKCOD's limitations as a democratic forum reflect entirely the extent to which the internet is still a primitive medium of political communication. Most people do not have access to the internet. Those who do tend not to use it as a politically interactive medium. Elites are scared of it. Most people over 30 are technically uneducated in its use. Web sites tend still to be techno-playgrounds, although user demographics point to recent changes, markedly in the area of educational usage. However sceptical one's assessment of the UKCOD initiative, or the relationship between ICTs and democracy in principle, it makes sense to suspend judgement until the new technologies become more firmly rooted in political culture. From a late twentieth-century perspective, neither technophobic dismissal nor hyperbolic enthusiasm are justified responses to these formative experiments in electronic democracy. More reasonably, principles of best practice for the future implementation of online direct deliberation projects can be outlined.

Open public forum

An open public forum, under the aegis of a neutral, non-partisan, public-service organisation, must exist for democratic online deliberation to be free from state or corporate control. Such a forum would conform theoretically to the ideal discursive conditions for a rational-critical public sphere outlined by Jurgen Habermas, although it would transcend the historically contingent exclusivity of the eighteenth-century coffee-house culture that embodied 'the bourgeois public sphere'. In relation to existing structures, the forum would conform most closely to that of the BBC, which has operated on the basis of a uniquely successful principle of public-service broadcasting, rather than dependence upon corporate sponsorship or government direction. A virtual public space could learn much from the public-service ethos of the BBC, but would, by the inherently decentralised nature of broadband digital discussion, be a more bottom up service: driven by its users, who would be both producers and consumers. Unlike the BBC, any attempt by the state to invade the autonomy of the virtual public space could not be brokered by arrangements between governing elites. Regulation would, of technical necessity, have to be transparent to all citizens. Given the economic imperatives of a capitalist society, no space, however public, is sustainable for long on the basis of voluntary effort. This is as true of parks and reference libraries as it is of electronic democracy services. If the political will exists to protect the integrity of public services, however, then, as in the case of the BBC, sponsorship arrangements need not undermine the independence of the service. The principle of independence is fundamental to the credibility and legitimacy of a public forum for direct deliberation.

Reliable online information

Online information must be current, multidimensional, fearless of complexity and always open to challenge. These may sound like a list of pieties from a 'mission statement', but they are important aspirations if online democracy is to rise above the level of well-intentioned amateurism. Much of the material to be found currently on the world wide web is outdated and poorly researched. Democratic discussion depends upon reliable information. Nothing would be worse than to establish an appealing forum for public deliberation in which citizens are provided with obsolete, incorrect or biased information.

One of the greatest problems of internet discussion so far is the tendency of the 'techies' to take control. Their priority is to enable users to reach information, but they are less interested in the quality of information provided. This is why any digital democracy service needs a clear editorial focus, aimed at providing high-quality content that is easily navigable and user-driven. Such provision needs to be multidimensional, utilising various forms of digital interactivity, from text to games and cartoons. When UKCOD developed the *Have Your Say* forum, with the help of the people of Trimdon, the aphorism of 'tabloid presentation, broadsheet journalism' was used as a guiding principle. In the medium of print news, flashy tabloid presentation tends to signal poor editorial standards, journalistic condescension towards their readers and a fear of complexity in the provision of information. Conversely, the broadsheets are journalistically more reliable, but not particularly user friendly. Newspapers have never succeeded in marrying the best of each form, but digital technology can. There is no reason to avoid tabloid-style front ends to web sites, with games, kids' areas and multidimensional variety, together with a core of worthwhile information. Web sites allow users to access information layer by layer on a need-to-know basis, so there should be room for both the simple precis as well as comprehensive analyses and availability of original source material. All such information, including interpretative commentary, must be constantly open to challenge by critical citizens. There must be scope to respond to analysis, to offer a different analysis (indeed, a different agenda for discussion) and to create links to other sources of information and commentary.

Inclusive public deliberation

Public deliberation must be inclusive, both at the point of access and in welcoming different forms of contribution to discussion. The much-rehearsed question of access is crucial to the formation of a truly democratic public sphere, but is ultimately a matter of public policy. Quite simply, 'digital democracy,' from which the majority of the population is excluded economically at the point of access, would be a political self-delusion. This does not mean, however, that until there is majority access all discussion of online democratic deliberation is redundant. The majority of the world's population have never made a telephone call, but that would be a poor justification for rejecting the need for public regulation of global telecommunications provision. Online democratic experiments must proceed on the assumption that most people will be digitally connected sooner rather than later. Those who have access, and are to obtain access, to digital communication should not be confined to forms of deliberation devised by previous media epochs. Broadcasters tend to give greater respect to the ideological over the experiential: ideology is for the 'heavy' political discussions, and experience for the 'soft' sounding-off outlets, such as phone-ins. This suits the structure of a one-to-many medium like broadcasting. Many-to-many communication permits experiential knowledge to return to its rightful place in the hierarchy of social communication. It allows people to discuss on the basis of what they know from doing as well as from contemplation. This does not mean that deliberation will collapse into an amorphous patchwork of individual experiences; on the contrary, people rarely choose to publicly recount their experiences unless it is to arrive at or support a point of view. Traditional media has been almost as cautious about citizens with organised views of the world as it has been dismissive of the political significance of experiential testimony. So, there should be every opportunity for citizens as members of interst groups or political parties to put their case without being accused of trying to take things over. An advantage of democratic interactivity is the range of forms that contributions to public discussion can take, from the anecdotal to the didactic.

Education for democratic citizenship

Democratic deliberation is wholly dependent upon the existence of a democratic culture. This is no different from voting: if enfranchised citizens choose to abstain or not think about how they vote, then elections lose their legitimacy and are easily manipulated by a professional elite, in line with Michels' iron law of oligarchy. So, basic to the creation of an environment conducive to democratic deliberation is education for democratic citizenship, a subject long neglected in the UK, but recently addressed with considerable perceptiveness by the Crick Committee (Crick 1998). Bernard Crick's long-standing concern to encourage 'political literacy' should now embrace media literacy, including a closer pedagogical relationship between the teaching of IT skills and the study of politics. Specifically, teaching is needed in skills of discussion facilitation and ways of articulating arguments simply and convincingly. School and university debating societies have tended to become ghettos inhabited by the pompous and the opinionated. Public debate in adult society is now an eccentric hobby; the days of open meetings in pubs and parks and on street corners are over (Coleman 1997). It was within such arenas of debate that many people first learned how to argue and form their own ideas (Ree 1984). These skills need to be relearned in the new context of cyberspace. One of the deficiencies of much online discussion so far, particularly in some of the news groups, has been the absence of hearing skills and the bad-tempered nature of many contributions. One might observe cynically that with the broadcast House of Commons as their deliberative model, it is hardly surprising that newcomers to public political debate lack good manners. It is a bigger issue than that, however: democracy itself is often seen as a game of tribal adversity and majoritarian head counting, in which all positions must be fixed and the object merely to win. There are other ways of conducting democratic discussion, and consensus can often be a more enduring value than victory in verbal battle (Barber 1984).

Links between citizens and their representatives

There needs to be a practical link between the voice of the citizens and the actions of elected representatives. In a direct democracy, this would take the form of delegates being mandated, accountable and recallable. Online voting is still a primitive and unreliable mechanism, and, as we have observed already, could be easy prey to electronic populism posing as enhanced democracy. Mature public deliberation deserves to be listened to by those in power, not because it is representative, but because it is thoughtful. Even a quite unrepresentative group of discussion participants is better than none at all, and from them representatives can learn much: about people's experience; about the communities to which citizens feel they belong; about the intensity of views held; and about why members of the public do or do not trust those elected to represent them. If all of this is ignored by the political elite on the grounds that 'it's just people talking', or because those entering into discussion do not constitute a demographic microcosm of society, then citizens will become less confident in their capacity to make a difference. This does not mean that they will stop deliberating – democratic opportunities are rarely cast aside once discovered – but that deliberation will proceed on the basis that representatives are remote and best overlooked. The example of the more populist trends in US talk radio in the early 1990s shows how this can happen and the extent to which popular disaffection can turn into populist disengagement from democratic discourse. So, it is to representatives' own advantage, as well as that of democratic culture as a political project, that direct deliberation by citizens not only takes place but is taken seriously.

Conclusion

Despite all of the limitations of the new media as channels of democratic citizenship, their role as a putative public sphere should not be neglected. Too much of the discussion about the revolutionary political potential of ICTs has been devoted to futuristic visions of direct democracy displacing political representation. Advocates of direct democracy have paid insufficient attention to the dangers of electro-plebiscites being appropriated by populist or demagogic forces. A more meaningful political contradistinction is between virtual deliberation – which has turned politics into a spectator sport while civic engagement has atrophied – and direct deliberation – a substantive condition of any healthy, participative democracy.

13 Participation, inclusion, exclusion and netactivism: how the internet invents new forms of democratic activity

Trevor Locke

Introduction

Community networks are developing in the UK, just as they have developed in North America and other parts of Europe. They represent an important departure in the provision of community access to information, telecommunications and IT resources.

Community networks are described as being people-oriented and place-focused. In the criteria set by the co-ordinating body UK Communities Online, such networks are characterised by some or all of these features:

- they offer a diverse range of information – not just 'official' material;
- they seek to involve all sectors of the community in their production and consumption; and
- they offer and encourage some level of interaction, from e-mail feedback through to full-scale conferencing.

Such networks can be run by a local charity or association, a regeneration agency, a private individual or by multiple partners. They often provide training and support to users, and free public access through a wide range of venues (such as libraries or community centres) (http://www.communities.org.uk).

It is true that communities of interest can and do exist on the internet as well as naturally in society. UK Communities Online has oriented itself to geographically bounded communities, even though it recognises that communities of interest will co-exist with these networks. Hence, it regards electronic networks as arising from pre-existing social and economic relationships and being part of the development and regeneration of geographical areas and their communities.

Debbie Ellen has formulated a Charter for Community internets in which she sets out a number of principles or values that characterise community networks. One of these principles is that of inclusion:

> commitment to the principle of social inclusion in the 'information society' for all (learn from each other networks that have found ways of providing access to the less well educated elderly people afraid of or uncomfortable with the technology, people on low incomes who cannot afford the hardware).
>
> (Ellen)

A principle often enshrined by these networks is freedom of access. In order to maximise inclusion, the networks are established in such a way as to allow the users to gain access to them at someone else's expense. Gaining access to the network is about gaining access to the opportunities that flow from it. Freedom of speech is another widely espoused principle associated with the way in which the networks are set up and operated.

The networks seek to involve all sectors of the community, allowing businesses to stand side by side with charities, the arts, recreation clubs and voluntary social services. It is frequently the users who develop the information that is placed on the network. Network developers, as a matter of principle, enable and encourage local groups and individual users to provide information, news and material for the networks. It is felt to be consistent with the general principles of community development that users should feel a sense of ownership for the networks in which they are involved. Debbie Ellen sees the outcomes of the networks as including:

- improvement of local democracy, through enhancing access to information and improved communication;
- improving communications between individuals and groups;
- improving opportunities for work and business;
- improving input to local planning and development;
- strengthening self help initiatives;
- supporting local organisations such as LETS schemes, credit unions, food co-operatives, volunteering or home working.

(Ellen)

David Miller of Sheffield University has considered community information networks (CINs), which serve the needs of users in a specific geographical area. Miller pointed out that early electronic information systems tended to be based either on video-text or on networked PCs. These were often under the control of some centralised authority, with decisions about content, where points of access should be placed and other key characteristics being made by network managers rather than by the users. He argues that the internet has allowed users to take control of the content and form of the information that they provide.

Miller distinguishes three types of network:

1   those initiated and controlled by the local authority;
2   those initiated and developed by the private sector; and
3   those initiated and developed by user populations.

There are a great many local information systems on the internet. For example, an index of web sites maintained by the London Borough of Brent includes 262 entries, the same number as the list maintained by the private sector company Tagish (figures taken in August 1997; new sites are appearing each week). There are many sites in the UK that provide information about local areas and that are maintained by private sector companies, such as local newspapers.

Even though bounded by a geographical area, community networks provide more than just information about a local area. Community networks are by their nature interactive, multifunctional, user-driven, and are a function of some broader regime of community development or regeneration. Whilst information provision might well be a key function of many web sites, it is the involvement of local people that determines that an initiative falls into the remit addressed by this chapter.

The network can be either a specially engineered intranet or one that is provided through the medium of the internet. Sometimes the network involves both of these, with gateways allowing access between the two in a controlled manner. Whilst some networks allow completely free access, some require users to register and thereafter log on to the network, even if they do not have to pay a registration fee. Sometimes there are areas on a network that are confined to local users and screened off from unfettered public access.

As Cisler has argued, in an early study of community networks:

Just as electrical systems began to transform urban and small town America a century ago, community computer networks will do so in the 1990s. The present situation is that few people are aware of the concept of community computing networks, any more than people understood much at all about electricity in 1890. Most of the attention has been paid to national research networks such as the internet and the commercial consumer services such as Compuserve, GEnie, Prodigy or business services such as MCIMail or Dialcom. On a local level thousands of electronic bulletin boards have been started by dedicated individual hobbyists, small business people, non-profits, corporations, federal agencies, other governments and educational institutions. What is striking about many of these ventures is that each group is relatively unaware of the activities by the other groups. Database providers such as Dialog and Mead Data stay out of the messaging business except for narrow uses; business mail systems are just beginning to make links to bulletin board networks, and the BBS networks are just learning about the internet.

(Cisler 1993)

Community networks and political participation

Community networks are creating additional platforms for political participation. The network provides a medium through which public and politicians can communicate, exchange information, consult, debate and gauge each other's opinions on the issues that confront them. It is a medium that replicates the more traditional face-to-face interactions and exchanges, as well as sometimes creating its own unique versions of political interaction.

It does this to the extent that users bring their issues to the network, seek to influence decision makers who are online, are willing to use its various platforms for debate or are open to being polled online. The internet – with its e-mail and web sites – is too often just an electronic replication of the printed media. Unlike the printed media, the internet is fully interactive, speeding up the exchange of views and information from say twenty-four hours to real-time (synchronous) communications through chat, video or audio.

Community Networks have grown around the world. Having been created first in North America and flourishing in Europe, they are now firmly established in the UK. As a reflection of their entry to the UK, Communities Online (COL) has been created to co-ordinate, resource and service the needs of this field. COL has an extensive web site of information about community networking (http://www.communities.org.uk). It aims to bring groups together, to inform the field and to encourage new community networks to come into being. Having secured funding, it now has a full-time director. COL provides a list of about forty community networks in the UK and Eire. One of the largest community networks in the UK is Hantsweb, which has over a quarter of a million pages of information and a countywide network that provides both a public media of communication and an intranet for the county council.

Access and inclusion

We know that only a minority of people have access to computers, let alone online computing, but we also know that access to the internet is rapidly increasing. It was reported that the number of PCs accessing the internet in the US increased from 15 million in early 1996 to 31 million in early 1997. Most internet access is made from home PCs, although access from work-based PCs is growing, increasing by more than 200 per cent between 1996 and 1997 (ISOC Forum 1997).

Whilst it is true that there has been an exponential rate in the growth of the internet, as measured by the amount of traffic and the volume of web pages, and a considerable increase in the number of people who access it on a regular basis, it is still by no means a mass media: it is limited to social, educational and economic elites.

The issue of access to technology, of inclusion in access and exclusion from it, is an important issue for politicians and educators alike. A recent report bears witness to this. The report (on ensuring social inclusion in the Information Society) was backed by IBM and strongly endorsed community networking as the way forward.

The Net Result, report of the UK National Working Party on Social Inclusion (INSINC), recommended two linked models to ensure social inclusion: local IT community resource centres and community networks. Between them, these initiatives provide well-organised information, access, training, and scope for electronic discussion forums. They enable citizens and community groups to become active participants rather than passive receivers of information. The report was launched on 24 June 1997 at the headquarters of IBM UK in

London. IBM supported the work of the independent working party, together with the Community Development Foundation.

So what role do these local networks play in distributing the opportunities and benefits of new technology? The aim of community networks is to bring the opportunities offered by ICTs, and the benefits they confer, to people who would not normally be able to gain access. They are oriented to people who are economically excluded from the personal ownership of such technology, to those who would otherwise be excluded from seeking information and from engaging in public communications.

Community networks have political implications, not least because they enhance and empower access to information. Already local and central government politicians (and local authority officers) have realised the potential of the internet for communicating with the public and offering them information. It is estimated (in 1997) that over half of all local authorities have some presence on the world wide web.

In Birmingham, the ASSIST project allowed people to discuss council policy issues, providing a channel of consultation between the public and their elected members. It enabled people to gather opinion and to engage in debate in ways that were entirely new. Some councils have experimented with their financial planning procedures by making council tax and spending plan information available on the internet. Financial information is ideally suited to internet communication: there is a lot of it, it is almost entirely documentary and textual, it constantly changes and it benefits from graphical presentation.

From the provider side, community networks are seen as enabling citizens to participate more fully in the formal structures of the national and local state. Paying officers to spend time answering public enquiries is expensive – a very resource-hungry service. The more that information can be made available on a self-service basis, the more cost-effective it becomes. Expensive resources like staff are better deployed on generating new information, implementing policies and evaluating them, rather than answering the telephone to tell Joe Public the same thing for the hundredth time.

One of the most frequently asked questions on the Edinburgh Public Information system was reported to have been 'Where can I get a refuse sack?' Answering that question has probably cost the local authority hundreds of thousands of pounds in staff time. Placing that information on the internet and on public access terminals released valuable resources to deal with other environmental issues.

Access and inclusion will be aided by both the provision of technology and by the intelligent deployment of that technology in the service of the public. Too often information is set out in a dull, uninviting and unimaginative way. Information producers seem to think that they can get away with lifeless presentations of text on computers that would never be allowed on more visual media. Fortunately, that is beginning to change. Information is becoming more multimedia, more animated, fun to use and engaging – making it more likely that the user will come back and use the technology again. Paper-based media are available to information providers. They have word processors and photocopiers, and thus the means of production are under their control on a DIY basis. The web, however, is a technically elite medium requiring specialised resources in its creation and specialised knowledge and skills to deploy those resources. In this regard, it is easy for professionals and technicians to gain a powerful hold on the internet. Fortunately, there is no shortage of people who want to liberate skills and resources for the benefit of the community.

Netactivism

In the US, the Rand Corporation completed a massive and seminal study called 'Universal access to e-mail: feasibility and societal implications'. The study considered the feasibility of making e-mail as commonplace as the telephone. In the concluding chapter of the report, the authors considered the policy conclusions and made a series of recommendations. They argued:

> We find that use of electronic mail is valuable for individuals, for communities, for the practice and spread of democracy, and for the general development of a viable national information infrastructure. Consequently, the nation should support universal access to e-mail through appropriate public and private policies.

A little later they observed:

> Individuals' accessibility to e-mail is hampered by increasing income, education, and racial gaps in the availability of computers and access to network services. Some policy remedies appear to be required. These include creative ways to make terminals cheaper; to have them recycled; to provide access in libraries, community centres, and other public venues; and to

provide e-mail 'vouchers' or support other forms of cross-subsidies.

(Rand Corporation)

Their evidence suggested that e-mail played a central role in the promotion and use of electronic networks. Evidence from the town of Blackburg in the US, where internet access was said to have reached some 60 per cent of the residents, suggested that the most popular function to be provided was e-mail. Residents' use of e-mail far outstripped that of surfing the world wide web.

The next step up from e-mail is the bulletin board, newsgroup and list server. For a few months last year, I subscribed to the US list server Civic Values, provided by the Institute for the Study of Civic Values (http://libertynet.org/{sim}edcivic/iscvhome. html). It was a very lively and active list, dropping more postings into my mail box each day than I could easily cope with. It was during my subscription to this list that I became aware of the concept of *netactivism*, primarily through the work of Ed Schwartz, a leading proponent of the application of the internet to political activism.

Ed's book *Netactivism: How Citizens use the internet* was published in 1996. The book described how:

> Electronic networks offer new channels for action from the neighbourhood to the national level. Now you can quickly find out what the government really does and organise around a cause or around a community using mailing lists, online debates, and web sites.
>
> (http://www.ora.com/catalog/netactivism/desc.html)

The flyer for the book astutely observed that

> this book is not a paean to the internet. It deals also with the real world outside the internet. Schwartz takes a hard look at what contemporary political movements need, whether they be about neighbourhood empowerment, ecology, children, or electing candidates to public office. The internet is not an end in itself, but a tool to wield in the constant job of organising people. This book discusses the roles of mailing lists, web sites, and community networks, and their relationship to traditional outlets for activism.
>
> (Schwartz 1996)

I would concur with these arguments, and believe that the internet is not an end in itself, it is a medium that is used and moulded like all other media to suit the ends of the users. It does not depersonalise users, rather people 'en-personalise' the internet.

Future trends and directions

The emergence in the UK of community networking is in itself a key trend that will influence access to information communications and technology. It is very likely that people will learn to use such facilities just as they have learnt to use the telephone, the broadcast media and computers. What drives users is their agendas, their desires, their anger, values, ambition, lust for power, public spirit, commitment to justice and equality, greed . . . all the things that have driven humanity for thousands of years. Technology may have changed since the times of the Greeks and Romans, the Egyptians and the Incas, but the underlying motivation and behaviour of its users has remained remarkably constant.

Some might argue that the essence of new technology will radically alter the way in which people think and act, that there are inherent properties within the technology that will bring about qualitative changes in human relationships and in social differentiation. It is argued that the internet is a great leveller – it depersonalises and allows anyone to do anything, irrespective of their race, age, sex or class. I doubt this. In fact, my experience suggests that this is decidedly not so. In a classic joke of the internet, a dog (seated at a computer) remarks to another dog that 'On the internet, nobody knows you're a dog.' My role as a chat room host on AOL leads me to suspect that whilst the internet is a cloaking device, in the final analysis the real person always shines through, if only dimly. As people become more fluent with the language of online chat, as they master its capacity for social communication, their real selves become revealed. The dog is sussed out, his canine properties finally being detected in his mannerisms, style and attitude. You can pass for a human being and fool some of the people some of the time, but at the end of the day you are still a dog and subject to doggy ways.

Although this might sound trite, it signifies an important principle for electronically mediated human transactions: the more you use the media, the more fluent you become. It's the same as speaking a language: the more you speak it, think in it, feel with it and live by it, the more difficult it is to detect that it is not your native tongue. No matter what kind of communications media is used, the more it is used the more fluent become its users. Just as language speakers become fluent in the spoken word, so signers become fluent with their medium of communication.

The internet is still relatively new and there is still a large proportion of people, even in advanced technological societies, who have not been on it. Television, however, is a technology that is omniscient: can there be even one sighted person in the UK who has not seen television? How many people hardly ever watch it? Even people who themselves do not own a TV, find they end up watching it at the home of a friend or relative. TV has become the technology that has penetrated everyday life and penetrated it the most deeply … even more than the telephone.

The advent of digital TV will, in my view, have a far more profound impact on everyday life for the majority of the population than the internet. It is very likely that the internet will continue to exist alongside the telephone and the wireless, but it will be, I suspect, the preserve of the literati: it will attract the devotions of a dedicated following, like citizens' band radio still does following the passing of its hey-day. Digital TV, however, will replace newspapers and the internet as the main infrastructure for the delivery of information. It will do everything that the exponents of the internet claim for their own medium, but it will do it better.

The internet is a wonderful thing, but the biggest barrier to its success is that you need a computer to get into it. More precisely, the biggest barrier to mass access to the internet is the keyboard. The keyboard is the artefact of the literary elite, the technically competent and the highly skilled. The mode of communication of the common person is the voice. Even the mouse is not a universally welcome tool amongst the IT-literati. Most people will cope with the remote control of their TV, providing it doesn't get too complicated. Within a few years, the keyboard will be as obsolete as the inked ribbon is now, as we learn to communicate with technology via our voices. That will open up technology and will be the most important development in providing access to technology.

TV has, up to now, been a largely passive device; digital TV, combined with a feedback loop with every box, will put access into every home. There is still something a little exclusive about the telephone. If that feedback can travel through the electricity supply, then that would open up interactive TV to universal enfranchisement. It will be possible to allow the individual to vote via their TV, ask questions and publish their opinions without needing specialised technologies. Interactive, digital TV carries enormous power because it gives everyone equal access to the means by which political persuasion is produced.

Even now, the media channels public opinion polling into the political arena. All opinion polls are, however, long-winded, manual procedures that must, in practical terms, utilise relatively small samples. TVs on the grid, however, will allow universal opinion polling and voting. A national referendum would be a routine event.

If we come back in ten years time to reconsider the impact of technology on democracy, we will hear little of the internet: it was just a passing technology, like the vinyl record and the audio cassette. It will occupy the same place in the history of technology as citizens' band radio. Its force and content will have been taken over by digital TV. Its interactivity and connectivity will find a much fuller life and vigour in the mass audiences of the TV set. Within about ten years, most households in Europe will have one box that will combine together our present domestic technologies of TV, telephone and computer. The implications of that for politics and democracy are quite profound.

14 The social shaping of The Democracy Network (DNet)

Sharon Docter and
William H. Dutton

Abstract

This chapter presents a case study of The Democracy Network (DNet) – one of the most innovative electronic voter guides geared to the American electorate (CGS 1998). An analysis of the motivations behind key technical choices in DNet's development highlights the significance of producers' conceptions of law and policy in shaping the technology of digital democracy.

The social shaping of digital democracy

Since the 1960s, scholars and policy makers have speculated about the way in which new information and communication technologies (ICTs), such as interactive television and the internet, might affect political participation and democratic institutions. Visions of teledemocracy focused discussion on the potential for ICTs to reform campaigns and elections (Dutton 1992).

Given the necessarily futures-oriented thrust of this work, much research concerning electronic tele- and cyberdemocracy has focused on utopian and dystopian arguments for (or against) the adoption of ICTs to promote (or protect) more democratic forms of participation. Some scholars have argued that electronic communication could improve the responsiveness of political institutions and allow for more direct citizen participation in public affairs (Sackman and Nie 1970; Sackman and Boehm 1972; Becker 1981; Williams 1982; Arterton 1987; Slaton 1992). Others have argued that electronic communication will be used in ways that diminish deliberation and thereby impoverish political debate (Laudon 1977; Abramson et al. 1988).

Most literature that examines the effects of ICTs on politics shares much in common with technological theories of media effects in the field of communication, where scholars have hypothesised numerous effects of the mass media on society (Innis 1951; Gouldner 1976; Eisenstein 1980; Carey 1989). Both literatures are rooted in technologically deterministic assumptions, where the inherent or designed-in characteristics of technologies are assumed to drive social organisation.

Ithiel de Sola Pool (1983: 5), for example, argued that the biases of ICTs, such as the microcomputer and online publishing, are democratising. He labelled these types of ICTs 'technologies of freedom', because their design fostered more decentralised structures of control over communication, but also he argued that excessive regulation could undermine the liberating potential of these technologies. Others have argued that the same ICTs can reinforce existing structures of power (Danziger *et al.* 1982), or support more centralised structures of communication, such as by disenfranchising the 'information have-nots' (Winner 1986; Schiller 1996).

Social shaping of technology (SST) research

Research concerning the effects and impacts of new media is exceedingly important. ICTs could influence access to political information, politicians, citizens and public services in profound ways, reconfiguring power relations within society (Dutton 1998). It is important to examine who benefits, and whether certain groups are likely to be left out of the political process (Schiller 1996; Loader 1998). Despite the significance of this issue, little empirical research has been conducted that examines the role of ICTs on patterns of political participation.

The shift away from impact research

In addition to examining the actual political role of ICTs, it is equally important to examine how electronic communications have been socially shaped by the producers and users of technologies. The design and use of technology, and the policies governing its use, will shape its political implications (MacKenzie and Wajcman 1985; Williams and Edge 1996).

More scholars have begun to examine technology not only as an independent variable shaping the social fabric of society, but instead favouring a more multifaceted approach, where social choices are assumed to shape technology, which, in turn, influences politics and society. For example, Pinch and Bijker (1987) argue that the design of technologies should not be treated as a 'black box' by social scientists, or as simply a neutral application and extension of scientific principles. Designs should be an object of inquiry, and viewed as the product of a history of social choices by producers, users and regulators (Pinch and Bijker 1987; Winner 1992; Williams and Edge 1996). Therefore, research should focus on the social – political, economic, cultural and legal – factors that shape technology, and reflect the social and institutional context in which they emerge (Bijker and Law 1992).

From this perspective, technology is inherently political in ways analogous to law and policy. Unlike policy decisions, however, technology is often designed without public scrutiny and debate among policy makers (Winner 1986; Dutton 1992: 518). In this way, technology can be viewed as being just as important to the social structure as laws, economic institutions or social beliefs (Winner 1986; Sclove 1992).

In ways analogous to the study of public policy decisions, theorists who examine the social shaping of technology assume that technology is not simply the result of rational product innovation, but arises from conflict and differences of opinion among a network of actors (Bijker and Law 1992: 8). Moreover, technical design features may advantage certain actors while disadvantaging others. Sometimes the conflicts and differences that shape technology are overt, at other times not apparent. As with policy, technical advantages can be intentional or unintentional, and can have unanticipated outcomes. Finally, it is assumed that social change and technical change occur together. To understand one fully, we must understand the other. Many technologists ignore the social, and many social scientists ignore the technical.

Legal models and analogies as a social force shaping technology

Prevailing law and policy are often claimed to lag behind technological change. Existing legal precedents and political-administrative traditions can also guide technological change, however, often by producers drawing analogies between the old and new technology. Law journals are replete with articles pertaining to how different legal models may be applied to the new electronic media, but little research has been conducted on how the law – and legal paradigms – shape technological choices. In the US, for example, conceptions of the First Amendment, and of how various First Amendment models apply to communication technology, could have a profound impact on how the technology is developed and eventually regulated (de Sola Pool 1983). If producers view a technology as something that places them in a legal position that is analogous to a speaker in the park, for example, then this could make a difference in what they believe is appropriate with respect to controlling content over this system, as compared to it being viewed as analogous to a broadcaster, or a common carrier, or a print publisher. Each analogy could lead to different design choices.

Approach of this study

Given the force of these SST arguments, and the potential significance of ICTs to democratic participation, few empirical studies have focused on the effects of teledemocracy (cyberdemocracy) projects, or on the social factors shaping the application of ICTs in government and politics (exceptions include Guthrie 1991 and Guthrie and Dutton 1992). This chapter seeks to contribute to the empirical understanding of social forces, such as laws and policy, shaping the design of cyberdemocracy, focusing particularly on the role of ICTs in political campaigns and elections. To gain a grounded perspective on these social factors, we focus on a case study of the most innovative electronic voter guide under development in the US, The Democracy Network (DNet). Specifically, our research seeks to advance an understanding of how conceptions of the First Amendment in the US, and how it applies to emerging ICTs, have shaped the design of cyberdemocracy initiatives. The analysis focuses on the social shaping of the design of a teledemocracy project, based primarily on in-depth interviews with its key developers that provide an understanding of the evolution of its design and the motivations behind key technical choices.

The Democracy Network (DNet)

DNet is one of the most innovative electronic voter guides geared to the American electorate. It provides an interesting example of the way in which democratic values in general, and free speech concerns in particular, can guide the design and implementation of a communication technology.

The Center for Governmental Studies (CGS), a non-profit organisation, designed DNet as a means for enhancing the quality of information provided about the issues at stake in political campaigns and elections. Its development was in part inspired by the optimism surrounding interactive TV in the early 1990s. Initial applications were all based on interactive video communication over ITV networks such as Warner's Full Service Network (FSN) outside Orlando, Florida (Burstein and Kline 1995). With the collapse of interactive cable TV (ITV) investments by industry in the mid-1990s, CGS shifted its attention to the rising media of the time, the internet and world wide web. DNet's web site was launched during the summer of 1996.

At its inception, DNet was conceived of as a video voter's guide for the viewers of interactive cable television. It was designed in anticipation of the next generation of public affairs television that would eclipse services, such as the Cable-Satellite Public Affairs Network (C-SPAN). It was to be interactive, community-oriented, and centred on the TV. Whilst it shifted to become more anchored on the internet and web, it remained focused on fostering more issue-oriented campaigns and more rational, issue-based voting, by providing improved information about the positions of all candidates on issues of the campaign.

Prevailing legal paradigms, particularly concerning the US First Amendment, as well as emerging technological paradigms (interactive TV) and conceptions of the rational voter, all shaped designs of this network. In addition, the faltering development of ITV, accompanied by the explosion of interest in the internet and web, had a dramatic impact on this model for how electronic media can be used to inform voters in the US, which has become a prototype for others round the world.

Motivations for launching DNet

DNet offers candidate- and issue-related information, such as candidates' issue statements, biographical data, and endorsements for candidates, and details regarding ballot initiatives in states like California, where the referendum has become increasingly popular as a means for more direct citizen participation in establishing policy. DNet was designed to create incentives for candidates to participate in the identification of key issues and in clarifying their respective positions. Additionally, it provided a forum for debate among candidates, as well as a medium for citizen-to-citizen and citizen-to-candidate communication, such as through 'live interviews' on the web.

DNet also represented an attempt to counteract the effects of disproportionate funding by candidates, by not charging for the provision of candidate information. The founders of CGS had been involved in public interest efforts to reform campaign financing rules, which bias elections towards those campaigns that can afford more paid advertising time on TV (Madaras 1997; Westen 1997). The internet seemed to offer an unprecedented opportunity to provide equal time, free from the cost and scarcity of broadcasting.

DNet targeted both national and local constituencies. Users nationwide could access information about the 1996 Presidential race. Along with this national information, users within the city of Santa Monica, California, could access information about local candidates and elections and state and local ballot initiatives (CGS 1997). In early 1997, users could also obtain information about local races within the city of Los Angeles, and plans were under way for DNet to provide content concerning elections in New York City and Seattle (Madaras 1997). By the run-up to the 1998 mid-term elections, DNet was expanded to cover elections in over nine states.

Features of DNet[1]

Features of DNet's design included both a broadcasting component, where communication was one-to-many, as well as an interactive component, where communication was many-to-many. The web site specifically included six distinct sections. A central broadcasting component included a menu-based system entitled 'On the Issues', where citizens could identify issues of interest to them and compare the issue positions of candidates. There was also a component called 'Candidate Info.', which provided biographical, contact and endorser information on the candidates, and 'Media', which allowed users to read stories in the press pertaining to the elections, by offering links to relevant online news.

The more interactive sections included a section on 'Ballot Measures', which provided users with official information pertaining to ballot measures such as summaries of the measures and arguments for and against them. This section was more interactive because users were given the opportunity to post their opinions about the measures and to read the opinions of other voters. A section entitled 'Your Views' functioned much like a bulletin board, where users could post comments and read the postings of others. In addition, chat rooms were available as well as a 'Match Poll', where users were provided with the opportunity to compare their opinions and positions with the positions of the candidates. This section also included the capacity for 'Live Interviews', where users could communicate directly with candidates or with experts concerning the election.

One such live interview was conducted on the eve of the November 1996 elections. State ballot experts from CGS answered questions about the ballot measures to be voted on in each public referendum. User reactions led CGS to plan the expansion of this facility (CGS 1997).

Finally, a section entitled 'Take Action' allowed users to send e-mail directly to the candidates. A form was also provided that allowed users to indicate a desire to contribute to, or volunteer for, a particular campaign. In addition to this interactive function, 'Take Action' also served a broadcasting function by allowing voters to find information of value to the election, such as polling places, voter registration information, and a guide on how to obtain absentee ballots.

A central component of DNet's design was its Remote Updating System (RUS) (CGS 1997: 37). Using this system, candidates enter personal identification numbers and passwords to allow them to update information, such as their position statements on issues, and their biographical, endorser or contact information. Through this system, they can also add issues to their election's issue grid, and get online help.

The issue grid

An issue grid creates a structure of incentives for opening up the campaign to a wider array of issues. If an issue already appears on the issue grid, a candidate can add their views on this issue. If candidates want to debate or state their position on a particular issue not represented on the issue grid, they can add the issue as well as a statement to the 'On the Issues' section of DNet. A red check mark shows that the candidate has stated his or her position on each issue. The candidates most recently up-dating or adding to their issue position statements are bumped to the top of the list of candidates, each of which is represented by a row within the issue grid. In this way, new information supersedes old information, and old issue statements are archived so that it is possible for a voter or journalist to examine how a candidate's position changed over time.

The issue grid, up-dated by candidates themselves, was important to DNet. Supporting the philosophy of the founders, the issue grid could hold candidates accountable for issue statements, as well as for their failure to address particular issues (Westen 1997). The issue grid, with its red check marks, makes it obvious whether or not a candidate has stated a position on any given issue.

In addition, the remote up-dating of the issue grid made it possible for the CGS to manage a large number of campaigns, despite limited staff resources. RUS enables content to be self-generating, much like content on other internet discussion groups. It would have required a far greater commitment of staff time for CGS to write, edit and manage candidate information, particularly as DNet expanded to cover elections in other cities and states (Madaras 1997; Westen 1997). Thus, remote up-dating supported the potential for a small non-profit to manage a nation-wide system.

The use of DNet

CGS found that DNet gained the participation of many candidates. A survey administered by CGS indicated that 'candidates liked the system, found participation to be fairly easy, and would have partic-ipated more fully using the Remote Updating System, if the technology had been available earlier in the race' (CGS 1997: 3). Moreover, DNet attracted a sizeable number of users, given the very emergent stage of internet use in campaigns and elections (Elberse *et al.* forthcoming). An independent web site research and measure-ment service estimated that DNet attracted approximately 3,000 users in less than a three-week period immediately following the launch of the web site. The most popular section of DNet was the issue grid, called 'On the Issues', where users could access candi-date issue statements and positions. The interactive pages of the web site, such as the chat rooms, 'Match Poll' and 'Your Views', also appeared to be popular among users (CGS 1997, 1998).

DNet received much publicity, including at least three stories in the *Los Angeles Times*, the major daily newspaper in the Los Angeles area. A story also appeared in the *Santa Monica Outlook*, and DNet was mentioned on local radio and cable programmes. In addition, the site received four online awards and generated several online news stories. National and international recognition led to its founder being involved in a variety of conferences and symposia on new media and politics. Its use expanded into the 1998 elections (Elberse *et al.* forthcoming).

Shaping The Democracy Network

A variety of social factors shaped the design of DNet. Legal models proved to be important, but broad conceptions of the user, particularly the kinds of media that would be most useful for reaching voters, also had a key role in shaping design.

Conceptions of the voting viewer

Both the ITV and web versions of DNet were created to address problems with conventional media, particularly US commercial television, and to build on the success of innovative public service television offerings in the US, especially the Cable-Satellite Public Affairs Network (C-SPAN). The founder of DNet, Tracy Westen, had championed the idea of creating a California version of C-SPAN and spent five years implementing this project (Westen and Givens 1989). The result was the California Channel, which broadcasts unedited footage of California State legislative proceedings via satellite to cable subscribers throughout the state. The California Channel does not editorialise in any way and provides viewers with the opportunity to see their state representatives in action.

Westen was convinced that TV has been the most effective medium for reaching voters. This led him to devote his efforts to the California Channel, and to the next generation of public affairs programming, which he saw possible with ITV. One problem with C-SPAN and its local equivalents, however, is that viewers cannot selectively tune into debate on issues of concern to them at convenient times (Westen 1997). Instead, the broadcast of legislative proceedings runs continuously and, therefore, may not be relevant to viewers' concerns at times of the day when a particular viewer is able to watch. CGS built on this problem as one advantage of taking C-SPAN another step, so that viewers could actively select from a menu of issues. In this manner, the information could be more immediately relevant to audiences. Rather than passively listening to legislative proceedings, viewers could be more actively involved in selecting areas of debate of greatest interest to them.

Like C-SPAN, the providers of DNet would not provide any editorial content. Instead, the content would be provided by the individual candidates, and DNet providers would be more akin to distributors of information. Designers, then, were able to use the emerging ITV industry (and later the web) as a means to correct a flaw with C-SPAN (Westen 1997).

An approach to inequities in campaign financing

Its developers also viewed DNet as a way to address problems with campaign financing. Westen and other principals of CGS are experts in the area of campaign finance reform. One CGS study into the California initiative process concluded that voters were not receiving the kind of information that they needed in order to make informed decisions on referenda (Stodder 1997). CGS recognised that although there is currently a proliferation of information about politics, the voters remain poorly informed on substantive issues of the campaigns. One reason is that most political communication from candidates to voters, particularly in US campaign advertisements, is in the form of thirty-second commercials, most of which fail to address many important policy issues facing the electorate. Because candidates are forced to spend large sums of money buying television time, they must focus their ads on the issue that will be the most salient to the voting public. This practice is the most cost-effective means of communicating with the electorate, and a rational strategy in the context of commercial TV. Ironically, this results in voters receiving less substantive information at the same time that more money is being spent on election campaigns. DNet, however, allows viewers to tune in to a broad range of issues. If a viewer is not interested in the issue addressed by the candidate, they can click to another issue (Westen 1997).

This was another concern behind the design of DNet – an effort to counter the effects of disproportionate fund raising (Westen 1997). In the US political arena of the late 1990s, the candidate that is able to raise the most money gains more exposure with the voting public (because they are able to purchase more television time). This is particularly critical since mere exposure to a political candidate increases the likelihood that a candidate will be favourably perceived. This is one reason why incumbents have such an advantage over non-incumbent challengers. In contrast, with DNet, participation is designed to be independent of financing; all candidates have the opportunity for equal exposure. Even candidates and parties with virtually no financing can get their message out to the electorate.

Technology shaping technology: the failure of ITV

The design of DNet was influenced by the technology of ITV. The promise of ITV emerged during the late 1960s in the US with the schemes for marrying cable and computer technology to wire cities

(Dutton *et al.* 1987). During the early 1990s, there was a resurgence of interest in ITV, with a great deal of press coverage on the promise of interactive applications (Burstein and Kline 1995). Communication experts believed that ITV would be the most important new technology to enter people's homes, and that it would be a trigger service for the 'information superhighway'. Industry leaders, such as Time Warner and TCI, along with some of the telephone companies, began laying the structure for fibre optic and hybrid fibre-coaxial cable networks, which would allow for two-way communication and which could potentially provide 500-plus channels of information and entertainment programming. Features such as movies on-demand, home shopping, games, and an increase in entertainment programming could be offered to viewers. Questions concerning the demand for such services were often dismissed in the enthusiasm surrounding new business opportunities.

Given the tremendous capacity available within an ITV system, designers of DNet recognised that information service providers would need to generate great amounts of content to carry over the system. They believed that they could convince the cable companies and telephone companies to carry their services (Stodder 1997). CGS began creating a prototype using actual candidates and ballot initiatives that would provide an interactive video voter's guide.

As discussed above, the principals at CGS liked the idea of communicating political information in video form, as they believed that viewers would find video programming more compelling than a text-only format. Voters would have the opportunity to see the candidates speaking for themselves, and this would give voters a good sense of the candidates as people (Madaras 1997). Moreover, the candidates appeared to have a similar conception of the voter – that communicating with voters through video would be more powerful than a text-only format – and, therefore, were willing to participate in ITV projects (Madaras 1997).

CGS enlisted the aid of a multimedia company to help design a prototype of their system. The original prototype included video candidate issue statements and answers to voter questions for the 1994 California gubernatorial and Secretary of State races. Also included was information pertaining to a controversial 1994 California ballot initiative on school vouchers, creating a system for families to use public vouchers to support their children's education at the school of their choice. Video statements from proponents and opponents of the initiative were included on the system as well as analysis from the State Legislative Analyst.

The system incorporated other media as well. For example, a campaign commercial against the voucher was included along with a truth box analysis of the ad by *The Sacramento Bee* (Stodder 1997). The system was menu-based, so that users could select information that they perceived to be most relevant to them.

When the prototype was completed in the fall of 1994, it attracted media attention, as it provided an example of the way in which the information superhighway could be used to provide public service information. The prototype was mentioned in major US newspapers, including *The Wall Street Journal* and *The Washington Post* (Stodder 1997).

Because the project had achieved a public presence, representatives from CGS were able to make contact effectively with the major leaders of ITV projects, including some of the Regional Bell Operating Companies and multiservice cable operators, such as Time Warner. At one point, it appeared that there were good possibilities of getting DNet installed in ITV systems planned by PacTel, Bell Atlantic, Nynex, US West, Time Warner and Viacom (Stodder 1997). By 1995, however, many companies began retreating from their ITV operations. They discovered that early demand for these services was not as high as initially anticipated, and questioned their long-term profitability. Most of those companies initially interested in the DNet prototype soon lost interest in the system.

One exception was Time Warner, which decided to proceed with its ITV Full Service Network (FSN) operations in Orlando, Florida. Representatives of Time Warner remained interested in DNet's participation and went ahead with plans to provide voter information concerning the November 1996 national elections. Representatives of Time Warner suggested that DNet designers work with Time Inc. New Media in New York, which was creating an interactive news channel called 'The News Exchange'. Time Warner suggested that DNet could be included as one part of this news exchange (Stodder 1997).

CGS began assembling content for the 1996 Presidential candidates. Whilst the initial goal was to have DNet up and running by the key primaries, multiple technical problems with the ITV system prevented DNet from being launched until August 1996, just before the Democratic and Republican Conventions. Whilst some of the information on DNet was out of date by this point, such as statements by candidates who had dropped out of the race, the system was up-dated to include information about Clinton and Dole.

Despite these problems, designers of DNet viewed its experiment with ITV operations to be a success overall (Madaras 1997; Stodder

1997; Westen 1997). There seemed to be high participation on DNet by candidates. Even incumbents, who are traditionally less eager to take political risks, participated in the system. Viewership was somewhat difficult to assess, and DNet was not actively promoted. CGS recognised, however, that they had successfully built the first interactive video voter system (Stodder 1997), and that whenever major industry leaders decide to move back in the direction of ITV, they would have the experience and knowhow to participate in the development of this technology (Madaras 1997).

The explosion of the Internet and World Wide Web

Despite the success of the Orlando experiment for DNet, Time Warner abandoned its FSN (Snoddy 1997; Dutton 1998). For the near-term, CGS recognised that ITV was not going to provide the wide dissemination of information they had originally anticipated. If DNet was going to reach a wide number of homes, then CGS needed to develop its application for those media available to voters.

By 1996, the explosion of interest in the internet was in full swing, and CGS began to realise that the web might provide a more viable system for video delivery, breathing new life into the CGS's vision (Madaras 1997; Stodder 1997). CGS began efforts to create a system with the key components of the ITV system, and to make this available on the internet, as well as over systems designed for web TV. Plans were begun to create a system on the internet that would provide community-based and national communication and information (Stodder 1997).

The role of ICT paradigms

The move from ITV to the web provides an example of the way in which technological paradigms can shape the development of a new technology (MacKenzie and Wajcman 1985: 8–13; Dutton 1996: 5–12). Within the scientific community, paradigms provide frameworks for knowledge by which data is ultimately interpreted (Kuhn 1970). They are 'time-tested and group licensed ways of seeing' (Kuhn 1970: 189), furnishing the analogies and metaphors that allow for the interpretation of new data and the research questions that are investigated. Problems that cannot be interpreted within the existing paradigm ultimately are not investigated. Eventually, new data that cannot be reconciled with the existing paradigm may lead to the development and shift to a new paradigm (ibid.).

Researchers concerned with the social shaping of technology have applied Kuhn's framework to the development of technology (MacKenzie and Wajcman 1985).[2] Rather than technology developing as part of a flash of scientific inspiration, technologies develop slowly, building upon existing technology and thus forming the basis for 'technological systems' (MacKenzie and Wajcman 1985; 12). Existing technology provides the model or exemplar within which new technology may be developed. As Donald MacKenzie and Judy Wajcman (1985: 10) argued: 'New technology, then, typically emerges not from flashes of disembodied inspiration but from existing technology, by a process of gradual change to, and new combinations of, that existing technology.' The finding that new technologies are based on older technologies suggests that the design decisions of older technologies will be very important as these form the basis for later design choices, which embed similar assumptions and biases (Johnson and Marks 1993).

In the case of DNet, ITV provided the paradigm for the delivery of information which was later applied to the web. Originally, candidate issues statements were included on the ITV system and viewers could select which statements they wished to access and compare candidate statements across issues. The original conception of DNet also included ballot information, and press information such as editorials. All of this information is included on the web. Moreover, as the capabilities of the internet and www have been enhanced, enabling easier access to motion video, CGS has sought to move DNet even closer to its earlier vision for ITV. In such ways, ITV provided a paradigm in terms of both format and content for the web site.

There are some differences between the ITV version of DNet and its web-based version. The original conception of DNet was almost anti-text, and key information was offered in video form (Stodder 1997). Given the textual nature of the web, text is a key component of DNet. However, like the ITV system, designers are working on incorporating more video onto the web. Whilst video currently is available over the web, the video must be downloaded and it takes users approximately eleven minutes to download clips. Efforts are being made to incorporate into the system a faster and more convenient method for users to access the video (Madaras 1997).

In addition, the web, through the use of bulletin boards and chat rooms, offers more opportunity for horizontal communication among users rather than the more one-way vertical patterns of communication from candidates to users supported by the mass-media. The voter-to-voter applications of the system appear to be among the most popular (CGS 1997). Finally, the web offered more flexibility than the ITV system, as candidates could instantaneously update statements and engage in debate through its RUS. In such ways, older technology has shaped newer technology.

Legal analogies leading new technology

CGS has been led by attorneys with expertise in communications law. One of the principals, for example, was a public interest lawyer and professor of communications law with expertise in free speech and First Amendment issues. This background contributed to free speech as well as other legal concerns having direct effects on the design of the technology.

Equal opportunities

One legal provision that had an impact on DNet was the 'equal opportunities provision' (Section 315) of the Communications Act of 1934. This provision applies to broadcasters and cable operators, and provides that if a station sells time to one candidate, the station must provide equal opportunities for all other candidates for the same office to purchase comparable time. Similarly, if a station gives time to one candidate, they must give comparable time to all other candidates for the same office. The equal opportunities provision had a particularly important role for two reasons. First, key developers of DNet had been advocates of the equal time provision in the broadcasting context, because it ensured greater fairness. It was important to the principals at CGS that this equal opportunities concern be applied to DNet, especially since the arguments opposed to equal opportunities in the broadcasting context seemed less applicable on the web. Thus, the structure of the system was built on the provision of equal opportunities for all candidates to participate. If one candidate provides an issue statement, then all other candidates have equal opportunities to offer competing issue statements or to create other issues for debate (Madaras 1997; Stodder 1997; Westen 1997).

Second, DNet can offer a system that is even more egalitarian than the equal time provision can be in the broadcasting context, as neither money nor space is necessarily a barrier to participation on the web. As noted above, in the broadcasting context, the equal opportunities provision applies to both free and paid commercial time. To the extent that one candidate has significantly more funding than another, cost provides a barrier to taking advantage of the equal opportunities provision, for candidates may not be able to afford comparable television time. With DNet over the web, however, candidates did not even need access to a computer to participate, as CGS made provision to enter even handwritten statements from candidates onto DNet (Stodder 1997).

Censorship

The equal opportunities provision shaped the design of the system in other ways, through its 'no censorship' provision. The equal opportunities provision of the US Communications Act provides that station owners cannot censor in any way the content of candidate television advertisements. The courts have held that this provision shields broadcasters from liability if one candidate libels another candidate in a television advertisement. Because broadcasters cannot control the content of the campaign advertisements, they are immune from liability (Farmers Educational and Cooperative Union of America v. WDAY 1959). The developers of DNet were familiar with this doctrine in the broadcasting context and saw it as applicable to their web site, realising that they must not control the content of any candidate statements, as this could open DNet to potential liability (Westen 1997).

Creating a system that ensured fairness to all candidates and that imposed a strict First Amendment ethic, in terms of not imposing any censorship, was also of value to the success of the system. It reinforced the developers' commitment to providing a system that was as neutral as possible and that avoided even the appearance of being partisan.

This was important for a variety of reasons. First, candidates would not want to participate if they perceived that the system favoured certain candidates or positions over others. One candidate, for example, expressed some hesitation about participating on the system because CGS offices were located in the same building as a candidate's campaign headquarters, creating the false impression that there was an organisational affiliation among them (Westen 1997).

Second, although CGS is a non-profit corporation, it is important that DNet obtain funding to support its activities. If DNet appeared partisan, then foundations and other potential funding sources would not be willing to provide support (Madaras 1997).

Finally, designers want various government home pages to create links to DNet. City governments, however, have very strict guidelines and cannot be perceived as sponsoring a candidate or point of view. For instance, CGS originally thought that DNet could be run by city clerks within cities around the country. It soon became clear to them, however, that city clerks were too concerned about doing anything that might appear partisan to be enthusiastic about administering such a system (Westen 1997). The city of Santa Monica, in particular, declined to offer a link to DNet because not all candidates participated on the system. Whilst all candidates had the opportunity to participate, only 86 per cent of the candidates chose to do so. Moreover, the city of Santa Monica has since decided to use its own web-based system, the Public Electronic Network (PEN), to support local campaigns and elections.

The First Amendment

CGS was influenced also by the type of free speech model that it viewed to be most applicable to DNet.[3] CGS principals, for example, recognised that the system was not akin to a common carrier, because designers drafted specific rules for communication, similar to something like Roberts Rules of Order in the electronic context. In this sense, DNet went well beyond the role of a common carrier (Westen 1997).

CGS carefully considered what the impact of particular rules would be. For example, they weighed whether candidates should be able to delete information.[4] They decided that candidates should not be able to delete old information; once a statement was made, it became part of the record of candidate statements, just as statements made in a newspaper cannot be deleted, even if those statements turn out to be inaccurate. Statements may be changed or corrected only by adding new statements (Westen 1997).

CGS also decided early on in the development of the system that they were not publishers of information, but distributors. As distributors and not publishers, DNet's developers were careful not to exercise any editorial control over content. By creating a system in which they distributed rather than published information, CGS attempted to position itself strategically in ways that would decrease any risk of liability.

Case law pertaining to electronic communications has established the principle that 'distributors' of electronic information may not be held liable for defamation, whereas 'publishers' may be held liable.[5] In the Cubby, Inc. v. Compuserve, Inc. (1991) case, a lower federal court held that Compuserve was a distributor of electronic information and did not exercise editorial control over content. As such, distributors of electronic information may not be held liable for defamation unless they 'knew or had reason to know of the allegedly defamatory ... statements' (Cubby, Inc. v. Compuserve, Inc. 1991: 141). Another federal lower court in Stratton Oakmont v. Prodigy Services Corporation (1995) held that Prodigy was a publisher of information because it created content guidelines and exercised some editorial control by providing services that instantly eliminated objectionable messages on its electronic bulletin boards. In light of this role, Prodigy could be held liable for defamation.

In 1996, Congress enacted the Communications Decency Act, which effectively overruled the Prodigy decision (CGS 1997). The Communications Decency Act states that online service providers may not be classified as 'publishers' and, therefore, are shielded from liability for defamatory statements made by users of such services (47 USC section 230 (c)(1)). In June 1997, sections of the Communications Decency Act were declared unconstitutional by the Supreme Court (Reno v. American Civil Liberties Union *et al.* 1997). The section of the Communications Decency Act shielding online service providers from liability, however, remained in effect. CGS (1997) knew that the Cubby standard also remained in effect, so that if online information service providers are aware of defamatory statements made by users, then they may be held liable for defamation.

More generally, CGS was well aware of this case law and statutory law which applied to online service providers and the distinction between 'publishers' and 'distributors' of information concerning liability (CGS 1996). They were influenced by this knowledge and recognised early on in the development of the system that they should not take on the role of publishers and, therefore, must not exercise editorial control. Instead, they saw themselves as distributors who provided a menu-based system for content provided by others (Madaras 1997; Stodder 1997; Westen 1997). In this instance, legal precedent had important impacts early on in the development of the technology.

Regulating indecency and obscene speech on the internet

The developers were also thinking strategically about how the courts would rule on the regulation of indecency and obscenity on the internet. CGS wanted to create a system of communication with as much uncensored speech as possible, as the principals wished to adhere to a strong ethic of free speech. Thus, the developers decided not to institute a policy where system operators would search for and delete indecent or obscene words. Rather than creating highly moderated discourse, CGS instead moved in the direction of providing uncensored discourse, whilst, at the same time, including a disclaimer that system operators may delete speech in order to protect themselves from liability. Along with recognising the importance of a free speech ethic, CGS recognised that they simply did not have the staff resources to institute such rules (Madaras 1997). Given these constraints, CGS imposed a 'Cubby-type' standard with regard to obscenity. Thus, whilst system operators were not instructed actively to search for obscene speech, if they became aware of obscene speech posted to bulletin boards, they would remove it from the system in order to protect themselves from any potential liability. As a practical matter, this issue was raised in only one instance, which did not require intervention from CGS.[6]

The regulation of campaign financing

Those who designed DNet were initially focused on content issues and liability, such as liability for defamation, but no candidate or voter raised the issue of defamation. Instead, candidates expressed concern about complying with Federal Election Commission rules concerning whether participation on the system might constitute an illegal corporate contribution. This became one of the primary legal issues tied to DNet (Madaras 1997; Westen 1997).

Whether a candidate's participation on DNet constituted an illegal corporate contribution was initially raised by President Bill Clinton's campaign staff in connection with the ITV project in Orlando, Florida (CGS 1997; Madaras 1997). According to Federal Election Commission (FEC) rules, it is illegal for corporations, even non-profit corporations, to provide services to candidates at less than the normal charge (CGS 1997). DNet's developers concluded that the system was a voter's guide, which was strictly informational and, therefore, fell within one of the exemptions to the FEC rules. The FEC had established very clear standards for determining whether a document constitutes a voter's guide. DNet was familiar with these rules and, as such, the system was designed to comply with the FEC standards. The FEC, for example, requires that voter's guides must direct questions to candidates. There was some question concerning whether or not the candidate's identification of issues constituted 'questions'.

Therefore, the system was redesigned so that participation came in the form of questions. Candidates, for example, were specifically asked to identify what issues they perceived to be important, and were asked to provide statements pertaining to particular issues (CGS 1997).

The issue of whether participation on DNet constituted an illegal corporate contribution was again raised by Clinton's campaign staff in conjunction with the web site. The FEC had ruled specifically that Compuserve and other internet service providers may not provide free internet access to federal candidates because this constituted an illegal corporate contribution. Members of Clinton's campaign staff were concerned that participation on DNet would also constitute an illegal corporate contribution. CGS developers countered that DNet was sufficiently different from Compuserve so as not to constitute an illegal corporate contribution. DNet did not, for example, provide free internet access, and candidates must use their own internet service providers to view DNet's web site. Moreover, DNet does not charge anyone for access, but merely provides a menu-based system for sorting the content provided by others (CGS 1997). Because of this, CGS argued, the service does not have any market value (Westen 1997).

Despite these arguments, the Clinton campaign declined participation on DNet's web site, arguing that they did not have time to review the legal arguments before the campaign. At this time, the Clinton campaign was already facing charges of engaging in illegal campaign finance practices. Thus, though not originally anticipated by designers, campaign finance rules had an impact on system design and policy, as developers were careful to design the system in such a way so that it would qualify as an exemption to the prohibition against corporate contributions.

Conclusion: law outpacing technology?

Studies of the social shaping of technology have argued that choices made by the developers of technologies are shaped by a variety of social factors. This is not to deny that technologies are embedded with inherent and design biases. Political communication via television encourages communication that is simplistic, visual, and that will immediately resonate with the voting public, often because of its emotional appeal. In developing DNet, its producers attempted to create a democratising technology that would be able to overcome some major limitations of the TV medium, be accessible to all candidates, and encourage voters to evaluate a fuller range of issues. DNet provides an example of technology as policy; technological design choices were made to shape distinct political and social outcomes, fulfilling the visions of its producers.

DNet came to be defined as a video voter's guide for interactive television, anticipating the next generation of public affairs television that would eclipse services such as C-SPAN. It was to be interactive, community-oriented and, above all, centred on the power of the TV image to connect with the voting public. It shifted to become more anchored on the internet and web, but remained focused on fostering more issue-oriented campaigns and issue-based voting.

Prevailing legal paradigms, particularly concerning the US First Amendment, as well as emerging technological paradigms and normative conceptions of the rational voter, who votes on the basis of issues, have shaped the design of this network. In addition, the faltering development of interactive cable TV systems, accompanied by the explosion of interest in the internet and web, had a dramatic impact on this model for how electronic media can be used to inform voters.

DNet provides another example of the way in which technological paradigms as well as public policy concerns can drive the development of technology. Moreover, because designers had expertise in the area of communications law, legal precedent had an important impact on the system's design. As such, legal issues did not arise downstream after the technology had been established.

Many legal scholars and social scientists assume that law rarely keeps pace with technology (Johnson and Marks 1993). They see the law applied to technology after its development to resolve emerging conflicts and litigation, as in the case of the Communications Decency Act. Issues raised over the conformance of DNet with campaign finance regulations conform with this expectation. With DNet, however, it was more often the case that legal issues were anticipated well in advance of the development of the technology, before the issues arose (such as in the case of liability for defamation). This study demonstrates that law can have an important role very early in the development of technology and therefore challenges more linear perspectives on the law and technological change. DNet could have been designed differently. Designers, for example, could have created a highly moderated system for discourse. Yet because designers were concerned about potential tort liability and embraced a strong free speech ethic (for both ideological and pragmatic reasons), designers declined to exercise editorial control and encouraged free and open debate in a manner accessible to the American public.

In addition, this case study suggests that the legal issues underlying the development of emerging forms of political communication are far from limited to models of content regulation, such as in the applicability of the First Amendment. Campaign financing, liability and other considerations such as copyright need to be more carefully examined in studies of the social shaping of digital democracy.

Notes

1 This section is based on use of DNet and various reports written by CGS, particularly a report on the launch of DNet's web site (CGS 1997).
2 MacKenzie and Wajcman (1985) credit Edward Constant (1980) with extending Kuhn's notion of a paradigm shift into the discussion of 'technological paradigms'. See also Guthrie (1991).
3 Discussions of the applicability of the First Amendment to emerging media include: Jensen (1987), Naughton (1992), Taviss (1992), Perritt (1993), Schalacter (1993), and Corn-Revere (1994).
4 Superficially technical issues, such as the deletion of information, often have profound political content. In this case, for example, revision of the historical record was a central theme of George Orwell's (1949) dystopian novel, *Nineteen Eighty-Four*.
5 For a discussion of liability in the context of electronic communications, see Becker (1989), Cutrera (1992) and Perritt (1992).
6 An indecent remark was made in a chat room, which at one time was part of DNet. However, since users could read only recent postings, the offensive remark was no longer publicly visible by the time CGS was able to investigate (Madaras 1997; Stodder 1997).

References

Abramson, J.B., Arterton, F.C. and Orren, G.R. (1988) *The Electronic Commonwealth: The Impact of New Media Technologies on Democratic Politics*, New York: Basic Books.

Agre, P. (1997) 'Computing as a social practice', in P. Agre and D. Schuler (eds), *Reinventing Technology, Rediscovering Community*, London: Ablex Publishing Corporation.

Aikens, G.S. (1997) 'American democracy and computer mediated communication: A case study in Minnesota', PhD thesis, University of Cambridge, also available at http://aikens.org.phd.

Allen, J. and Hamnett, C. (eds) (1995), *A Shrinking World? Global Unevenness and Inequality*, New York: Open University Press.

American Civil Liberties Union (1996) 'Appellee brief in Reno v. ACLU', no. 96–511, available at: http://www.aclu.org/court/renovaclu.html.

Anckar, D. (1982) 'A definition of democracy', *Scandinavian Political Studies*, 5, 3, pp. 217–235.

Ansolabehere, S. (1994) 'Does attack advertising demobilize the electorate?', *American Political Science Review*, 88, 4, pp. 829–838.

Arendt, H. (1958) *The Human Condition*, Chicago: University of Chicago Press.

Arendt, H. (1977) *Between Past and Future*, New York: Penguin.

Arterton, C. (1987) *Teledemocracy: Can Technology Protect Democracy?*, Newbury Park, CA: Sage.

Barber, B. (1984) *Strong Democracy: Participatory Politics for a New Age*, Berkeley: University of California Press.

Barber, B. (1995) *Jihad vs. McWorld*, New York: Times Books.

Barlow, J.P. (1996) 'Declaration of the independence of cyberspace', *Cyber-Rights Electronic List*, 8 February.

Beamish, A. (1995) '*Communities online: Community based computer networks*', unpublished masters thesis, MIT, Cambridge, MA.

Becker, G.S. (1983) 'A theory of competition among pressure groups for political influence', *Quarterly Journal of Economics*, 98, 3, pp. 371–399.

Becker, L.E. (1989) 'The liability of computer bulletin board operators for defamation posted by others', *Connecticut Law Review*, 22, pp. 203–272.

Becker, T. (1981) 'Teledemocracy: Bringing power back to the People', *Futurist*, December, pp. 6–9.

Becker, T. (1998) 'Governance and electronic innovation: A clash of paradigms', *Information, Communication and Society*, 1, 3 pp. 339–343.

Bellah, R. *et al.* (1985) *Habits of the Heart*, Berkeley: University of California Press.

Bellamy, C. and Taylor, J. (1998) *Governing in the Information Age*, London: Open University Press.

Benedikt, M. (ed.) (1991) *Cyberspace: First Steps*, Cambridge, MA: MIT Press.

Berry, J.M. (1989) *The Interest Group Society*, 2nd edition, Glenview, Ill.: Scott Foresman.

Berry, J.M., Portney, K.E. and Thomson, K. (1993) *The Rebirth of Urban Democracy*, Washington, DC: Brookings Institution Press.

Bijker, W.E. and Law, J. (1992), *Shaping Technology/Building Society: Studies in Sociotechnical Change*, Cambridge, MA: MIT Press.

Bimber, B. (1996). 'The internet and political transformation', available at http://www.sscf.ucsb.edu/~survey1/

Bird, J. (1996) 'It's all IT to me!', *Management Today*, June, pp. 78–81.

Blair, A. (1996) 'Switch on the bright ideas', *Guardian*, May 27, p. 13.

Blakely, E.J. and Snyder, M.G. (1997) *Fortress America: Gated Communities in the United States*, Washington, DC: Brookings Institution Press.

Blumler, J. and Gurevitch, M. (1996) *The Crisis in Public Communication*, London: Routledge.

Bonchek, M.S. (1995) *Grassroots in Cyberspace: Using Computer Networks to Facilitate Political Participation*, paper presented at the Midwest Political Science Association Meeting, available at http://www.ai.mit.edu/people/msb/pubs/grassroots.html

Budge, I. (1996) budge://the.new.challenge.of.direct.democracy/, Cambridge: Polity Press.

Bulos, M. and Sarno, C. (1996) *Codes of Practice and Public Closed Circuit Television Systems: A Report for the Local Government Information Unit*, School of Urban Development and Policy, Southbank University, London: Local Government Information Unit.

Burgelman, J. (1994) 'Assessing information technologies in the information society', in S. Splichal, A. Calabrese and C. Sparks (eds) *Information Society and Civil Society*, West Lafayette: Purdue University Press.

Burke, E. (1846–8) *Collected Works*, London.

Burstein, D. and Kline, D. (1995) *Road Warriors: Dreams and Nightmares Along the Information Highway*, New York: Dutton.

Bush, V. (1955) 'As we think', *The Atlantic Monthly*.

Calhoun, C. (1994) 'Introduction: Habermas and the public sphere', in C. Calhoun (ed.), *Habermas and the Public Sphere*, Cambridge, MA: MIT Press.

Campbell, A. *et al.* (1960) *The American Voter*, New York: Wiley.

Carey, J. (1989) *Communication as Culture*, Boston: Unwin Hyman.

Castells, M. (1995) *The Informational City*, Oxford: Blackwell.

Castells, M. (1997) *The Rise of the Network Society Volume 2: The Power of Identity*, Oxford: Blackwell.

CGS (1996) *DNet Libel Memorandum*, Los Angeles: CGS, October 22.

CGS (1997) *Democracy Comes to the internet: Report on the Launch of The Democracy Network Web Site During the November 1996 Elections*, Los Angeles: CGS.

CGS (1998) The Democracy Network at: http://www.democracynet.org

Chen, K. (1992) *Political Alienation and Voting Turnout in the United States, 1960–1988*, New York: Mellen Research University Press (based on doctoral dissertation, Columbia University).

Chomsky, N. interviewed by Rosie X and Chris Mountford, 'That's a little more information than I need to know, or informations anarchy and the plight of the igno-rant', available at http://www.next.com.au/spyfood/geek-girl/002manga/chomsky.html

Cisler, S. (1993) *Community Computer Networks: Building Electronic Greenbelts*, on the web at http://bliss.berkeley.edu/impact/speakers/cisler/cisler-talk.html

Coleman, J.S. (1988) 'Social capital in the creation of human capital', *American Journal of Sociology*, 94 (Supplement), S95 S120.

Coleman, S. (1997) *Stilled Tongues: From Soapbox to Soundbite*, London: Porcupine Press.

Coleman, S. (1998) 'BBC Radio's *Talkback* phone-in: Public feedback in a divided public space', *Javnost/the public*, 2.

Coleman, S. (1999) 'BBC Election Call: A democratic public forum?', Hansard Society.

Coleman, S., Taylor, J. and Donk, W.B.H.J. van de (1999) *Parliament in the Age of the Internet*, Oxford: Oxford University Press.

Commission on Freedom of the Press (1947) *A Free and Responsible Press: A General Report on Mass Communication*, Chicago: University of Chicago Press.

Communications Act of 1934, as amended 47 U.S.C. section 223 et seq. and 315 *et seq.*

Connolly, W. (1995) *The Ethos of Pluralization*, Minneapolis: University of Minnesota Press.

Constant, E.W. II (1980) *The Origins of the Turbojet Revolution*, Baltimore and London: Johns Hopkins.

Corbato, F. and Fano, R. (1966) 'Time sharing on computers', in authors *Information: A Scientific American Book*, San Francisco: Scientific American.

Corn-Revere, R. (1994), 'New technology and the First Amendment: Breaking the cycle of repression', *Hastings Comm/Ent Law Journal*, 17, pp. 247–345.

Creighton, J.L. (1995) 'Trends in the field of public participation in the United States', *Interact: The Journal of Public Participation*, 1, 1, pp. 7–23.

Crick, B. (1998) *Education for Citizenship and the Teaching of Democracy in Schools*, London: QCA.

Crow, G. and Allan, G. (1994) *Community Life: An Introduction to Local Social Relations*, London: Harvester Wheatsheaf.

Cubby, Inc. v. Compuserve, Inc., 776F. Supp. 135 (S.D.N.Y. 1991)

Cutrera, T.A. (1992), 'Computer networks, libel and the first amendment', *Computer Law Journal*, 11, pp. 555–583.

Dahl, R. (1970) *After the Revolution: Authority in a Good Society*, New Haven: Yale University Press.

Dahlgren, P. (1991) 'Introduction', in P. Dahlgren and C. Sparks (eds), *Communication and Citizenship*, London: Routledge.

Danziger, J.N., Dutton, W.H., Kling, R. and Kroemer, K.L. (1982) *Computers and Politics*, New York: Columbia University Press.

Davies, M. (1990) *City of Quartz: Excavating the Future in Los Angeles*, London: Vintage.

Davies, S. (1996) *Big Brother: Britain's web of Surveillance and the New Technological Order*, London: Pan Books.

De Tocqueville, A. (1945) *Democracy in America* (Volume 2), New York: Vintage Books.

DEMOS (1997) *Chain Reaction: Tackling Network Poverty*, London: DEMOS.

Dennis, A.R. and Valacich, J.S. (1993) 'Computer brainstorms: More heads are better than one', *Journal of Applied Psychology*, 78, pp. 531–537.

Derrida, J. (1992) *The Other Heading: Reflections on Today's Europe*, translated by P.A. Brault and M.B. Naas, Bloomington: Indiana University Press.

Dewey, J. (1927) *The Public and Its Problems*, London: Allen & Unwin.

Dickinson, H.T. (1977) *Liberty and Property: Political Ideology in Eighteenth Century Britain*, London: Weidenfeld & Nicolson.

Dienel, P.C. (1991) *Die Planungszelle*. 2, Aufl. Opladen: Westdt. Verlag.

Dijk, J. van (1996) 'Models of democracy: Behind the design and use of new media in politics', in *Javnost/The Public*, 3, 1, pp. 43–56.

Dionne, E.J. Jr. (1991) *Why Americans Hate Politics*, New York: Simon & Schuster.

Donk, W.B.H.J. van de and Tops, P.W. (1995) 'Orwell or Athens? Informatization and the future of democracy. A review of the literature', in W.B.H.J. van de Donk et al., *Orwell in Athens: A Perspective on Informatization and Democracy*, Amsterdam: IOS Press.

Donk, W.B.H.J. van de, Snellen, I.Th.M. and Tops, P.W. (1995) *Orwell in Athens: A Perspective on Informatization and Democracy*, Amsterdam: IOS Press.

Downs, A. (1957) *Economic Analysis of Democracy*, New York: Harper & Row.

Dunn, J. (1990) Interpreting Political Responsibility, Cambridge: Polity Press.

Dunleavy, P. (1991) *Democracy, Bureaucracy and Public Choice: Economic Explanations in Political Science*, London: Harvester Wheatsheaf.

Dunsire, A. (1994) 'Modes of governance', in J. Kooiman (ed.), *Modern Governance*, London: Sage.

Dutton, W.H. (1992) 'Political science research on teledemocracy', *Social Science Computer Research*, 10, 4, pp. 505–522.

Dutton, W.H. (1996) 'Network rules of order: Regulating speech in public electronic fora', *Media, Culture and Society*, 18, pp. 269–290.

Dutton, W.H. (ed.) (1996) *Information and Communication Technologies: Visions and Realities*, Oxford: Oxford University Press.

Dutton, W.H. (1998) *Society on the Line: Information Politics in the Digital Age*, Oxford: Oxford University Press.

Dutton, W.H., Blumler, J.G. and Kraemer, K.L. (eds) (1987) *Wired Cities: Shaping the Future of Communications*, Boston: G.K. Hall.

Dyson, E. (1997) *Release 2.0: A Design for Living in the Digital Age*, New York: Broadway.

Eisenstein, E.L. (1980), 'The emergence of print culture in the West', *Journal of Communication*, 30, pp. 99–105.

Ekos Research Associates (1998) Rethinking Citizen Engagement. Wave 1 Results, paper presented at the Privy Council Office-Canadian Centre for Management Development Seminar Series in Ottawa 17 April.

Elberse, A., Hale, M. and Dutton, W.H. (forthcoming) 'Network democracy', in K. Hacker and J. van Dijk (forthcoming), *Virtual Democracy: Issues in Theory and Practice*, Thousand Oaks, CA: Sage.

Ellen, D. on the web at http://www.communities.org.uk

Elshtain, J.B. (1982) 'Democracy and the QUBE tube', *The Nation*, 234, pp. 108–110.

Engelman, R. (1990) 'The origins of public access cable television, 1966–72', *Journalism Monographs*, No. 123.

Etzioni, A. (1988) *The Moral Dimension: Toward a New Economics*, New York: The Free Press.

European Union (1996) *Living and Working in the Information Society*, Brussels: European Union.

Fallow, J. (1996) *Breaking the News: How the Media Undermine American Democracy*, Farmers Educational and Cooperative Union of America v. WDAY, 360 U.S. 525, 79 S.Ct. 1302 (1959)

Featherly, K. 'MN-POLITICS, don't post'. Channel 4000, available at http://www.wcco.com/news/stories/news-970321-011624.html

Feldman, T. (1997) *An Introduction to Digital Media*, New York: Routledge.

Finer, S.E. (1984) 'The decline of party?', in V. Bogdanor (ed.) *Parties and Democracy in Britain and America*, New York: Praeger.

Fishkin, J. (1991) *Democracy and Deliberation: New Directions for Democratic Reform*, New Haven: Yale University Press.

Fishkin, J. (1992) 'Beyond teledemocracy: 'America on the line', *The Responsive Community*, 2, pp. 13–19.

Fishkin, J. (1995) *The Voice of the People: Public Opinion and Democracy*, New Haven: Yale University Press.

Fotopoulos, T. (1997) *Towards an Inclusive Democracy*, London: Cassell.

Foucault, M. (1977) *Discipline and Punish: The Birth of the Prison*, London: Allen Lane.

Fox, C.J. and Miller, H.T. (1995) *Postmodern Public Administration: Toward Discourse*, Thousand Oaks, CA: Sage.

Fyfe, N.R. and Bannister, J. (1996) 'City watching: Closed circuit television in public spaces', *Area*, 28, 1, pp. 37–46.

Gallagher, T. 'An early history of UK Citizen's Online Democracy', available at http://www.netnexus.org/library/papers/gallagher.htm

Gandy, O. (1994) *The Panoptic Society*, Boulder, CO: Westview.

Garnham, N. (1994) 'The media and the public sphere', in C. Calhoun (ed.), *Habermas and the Public Sphere*, Cambridge, MA: MIT Press.

Gates, B. (1995) *The Road Ahead*, London: Penguin.

Giddens, A. (1979) *Central Problems in Social Theory: Action, Structure and Contradiction in Social Analysis* Berkeley and Los Angeles: University of California Press.

Giddens, A. (1985) *The Nation-State and Violence*, Cambridge: Polity Press.

Giddens, A. (1994a) *New Rules of Sociological Method*, Cambridge: Polity Press.

Giddens, A. (1994b) *The Consequences of Modernity*, Cambridge: Polity Press.

Giddens, A. (1998) 'After the left's paralysis', *New Statesman*, May pp. 18–21.

Gouldner, A.W. (1976) *The Dialectic of Ideology and Technology*, New York: Seabury Press.

Government of Canada Internet Strategy in Government of Canada Internet Guide, available at http://www.tbs-sct.gc.ca/

Government Use of the Internet, G7 Governments Online and International Council for Information Technology in Government, available at http://www.open.gov.uk/govoline/latest1.htm

Graham, S. (1996) 'CCTV – Big brother or friendly eye in the sky?', *Town and Country Planning*, 65, 2, pp. 57–60.

Graham, S., Brooks, J. and Heery, D. (1996) 'Towns on television: Closed circuit television surveillance in British towns and cities', *Local Government Studies*, 22, 3, pp. 1–27.

Granovetter, M. (1982) 'Economic action and social structure: The problem of embeddedness', *American Journal of Sociology*, 91, 3, pp. 489, as quoted in Putnam, R. (1993) *Making Democracy Work*, Princeton: Princeton University Press.

Groper, R. (1996) 'Electronic mail and the reinvigoration of American democracy', *Social Science Computer Review*, 14, pp. 157–168.

Grossman, L.K. (1995) *The Electronic Republic: Reshaping Democracy in the Information Age*, New York: Viking.

Guthrie, K., *et al.* (1990) *Communication Technology and Democratic Participation: PENers in Santa Monica.* Paper presented at the Association of Computer Macinery's (ACM) Conference on 'Computers and the Quality of Life' Washington, DC September 12.

Guthrie, K.K. (1991) 'The politics of citizen access technology: The development of communication and information utilities in four cities', unpublished
PhD dissertation, Los Angeles, CA: The Annenberg School for Communication, University of Southern California.

Guthrie, K.K. and Dutton, W.H. (1992) 'The politics of citizen access technology: The development of public information utilities in four cities',
Policy Studies Journal, 20, 4, pp. 574–597.

Habermas, J. (1975) *Legitimation Crisis*, translated by T. McCarthy, Boston:
Beacon Press.

Habermas, J. (1984 [1981]) *The Theory of Communicative Action, Volume
One: Reason and the Rationalization of Society*, translated by T.
McCarthy, Boston: Beacon Press.

Habermas, J. (1987 [1985]) *The Theory of Communicative Action, Volume
Two: Lifeworld and System: A Critique of Functionalist Reasoning*, translated by T. McCarthy, Boston: Beacon Press.

Habermas, J. (1989) *The Structural Transformation of the Public Sphere:
An Inquiry into a Category of Bourgeois Society*, Cambridge: Polity
Press.

Habermas, J. (1990 [1983]) *Moral Consciousness and Communicative
Action*, translated by C. Lenhardt and S.W. Nicholsen, Cambridge, MA:
MIT Press.

Habermas, J. (1994a) 'Concluding remarks,' in C. Calhoun (ed.), *Habermas
and the Public Sphere*, Cambridge, MA: MIT Press.

Habermas, J. (1994b) 'The emergence of the public sphere', in J. Habermas,
The Polity Reader in Cultural Theory, Cambridge: Polity Press

Habermas, J. (1996 [1992]) *Between Facts and Norms: Contributions to a
Discourse Theory of Law and Democracy*, trans. W. Rehg, Cambridge,
MA: MIT Press.

Hacker, K. and van Dijk, J. (forthcoming) *Virtual Democracy: Issues in
Theory and Practice*. Thousand Oaks, CA: Sage.

Hacker, K. and Todino, M. (1996) 'Virtual democracy at the Clinton White
House: An experiment in electronic democracy', *Javnost/the public*, 3, 1,
pp. 71–86.

Halam-Baker, P. Message to intercog@ccta.gov.uk

Hale, M. (1997) 'California cities and the world wide web', unpublished
masters thesis, University of Southern California.

Hale, P. and Sourani, L. (1998) 'Virtual workshop on regulatory efficiency:
An innovative approach to consultations', *Canadian Institute of Mining,
Metallurgy and Petroleum (CIM) Bulletin* April 1998, available at
http://www.nrcan.gc.ca/mms/cim/virtual.htm

Hall, S. and Jacques, M. (eds) (1990) *New Times*, London: Lawrence &
Wishart.

Hall, S., Held, D. and McGrew, T. (eds) (1993) *Modernity and its Futures*,
Cambridge: Polity Press in association with Open University.

Halpern, D. (1998) 'Social capital, exclusion and the quality of life: Toward
a causal model and policy implications', Nexus Briefing Document

Hammer, M. (1990) 'Reengineering work: Don't automate, obliterate', Harvard Business Review, 64, 4, pp. 104–118.

Hardt, H. (1996) 'The making of the public sphere: Class relations and communication in the United States', *Javnost/the public*, 3, 1, pp. 7–23.

Harvey, D. (1989) *The Conditions of Postmodernity*, Cambridge: Polity Press.

Held, D. (1987) *Models of Democracy*, Cambridge: Polity Press.

Held, D. (1993) *Political Theory and the Modern State*, Cambridge: Polity Press.

Held, D. (1996) *Models of Democracy* (2nd edn) Cambridge: Polity Press.

Hobsbawm, E. (1996) 'If the truth be told', *Guardian*, 20 June p. 17.

Hoggett, P. (1990) *Modernisation, Political Strategies and the Welfare State*, Bristol: SAUS.

Holderness, M. (1998) 'Who are the world's information poor?', in Holderness, M., *The Cyberspace Divide: Equality, Agency and Policy in the Information Society*, London: Routledge.

Holmes, D. (ed.) (1997) *Virtual Politics: Identity and Community in Cyberspace*, London: Sage.

Home Office (1994) *Closed Circuit Television: Looking Out For You*, London: HMSO.

Home Office (1995a) *Closed Circuit Television: Winners by Government Regional Offices*, London: Home Office.

Home Office (1995b) *Preventing Crime Into the Next Century: Michael Howard*, News Release, 22 November, London: Home Office.

Home Office (1996a) *British Crime Survey*, London: Home Office.

Home Office (1996b) *Closed Circuit Television Challenge Competition 1996/97: Successful Bids*. London: Home Office.

Home Office (1997) *Closed Circuit Television Challenge 3 Competition 1997/98: Successful Bids*, Crime Prevention Agency, London: Home Office.

Home Office (1998) *CCTV Challenge Competition 1998/99: List of Winners by Region*, Home Office Press Release, 17 June, London: Home Office.

Honess, T. and Charman, E. (1992) *Closed Circuit Television in Public Places: Its Acceptability and Perceived Effectiveness*, Home Office Police Research Group, Crime Prevention Unit Series, Paper No. 35, London: Home Office.

Horrocks, I., Hoff, J. and Tops, P. (1999) *Democratic Governance and New Technology: Technologically Mediated Innovations in Political Practice in Western Europe*, London: Routledge.

House of Lords (1998) *Digital Images as Evidence*, Select Committee on Science and Technology, Fifth Report, London: HMSO.

Huckfeldt, R. and Sprague, J. (1995) *Citizens, Politics, and Social Communication*, Cambridge: Cambridge University Press.

Hunter, C.D. (1997) *Interaction and Political Party Web Pages*, paper presented to Eastern States Communication Association Conference, Baltimore.

Innis, H. (1951) *The Bias of Communication*, Toronto: University of Toronto Press.

Institute for the Study of Civic Values on the web at http://libertynet.org/~edcivic/iscvhome.html

Isenmann, S. and Reuter, W.D. (1996) 'Ist IBIS in der Praxis anwendbar? and Einige Erfahrungen und Folgerungen', in H. Krcmar, H. Lewe and G. Schwabe (eds), *Herausforderung Telekooperation*. Fachtagung DCSCW, Stuttgart-Hohenheim, 30 September–2 October, Berlin: Springer.

ISOC Forum (1997) 3, 7.

ISPO (1998) *Basic Indicators*, available at http://www.ispo.cec.be/Basic

Janda, K. (1978) 'A microfilm and computer system for analyzing comparative politics literature', in G. Gerbner *et al.* (eds), *The Analysis of Communication Content*, Huntington, NY: Robert E. Krieger Publishers, pp. 407–435.

Jensen, E.C. (1987), 'An electronic soapbox: Computer bulletin boards and the First Amendment', *Federal Communications Law Journal*, 39, pp. 217–258.

Johnson, D.R. and Marks, K.A. (1993) 'Mapping electronic data communications onto existing legal metaphors: Should we let our conscience (and our contracts) be our guide?', *Villanova Law Review*, 38, pp. 487–515.

Joseph Rowntree Reform Trust (1996) State of the Nation Poll, London, 1.

Kahn, F.J. (ed.) (1973) *Documents of American Broadcasting*, New York: Appleton-Century-Crofts.

Katz, J. (1997) 'The digital citizen', *Wired* 5, pp. 68–77.

Katz, R.S. (1990) 'Party as linkage: A vestigial function?', *European Journal of Political Research*, 18, pp. 143–161.

Kelly, C. (1989) 'Political identity and perceived intragroup homogeneity', *British Journal of Social Psychology*, 28, pp. 239–250.

Kiesler, S. and Sproull, L. (1992) 'Group decision making and communication technology', *Organizational Behavior and Human Decision Making* 52, pp. 96–123.

Kimber, R. (1989) 'On democracy', *Scandinavian Political Studies*, 12, 3, pp. 199–219.

Kirchheimer, O. (1966) 'The transformation of the Western European party system', in J. Lapalombara and M. Weiner (eds), *Political Parties and Political Developments*, Princeton: Princeton University Press.

Kraemer, K.L. and King, J.L. (1988) 'Computer-based systems for co-operative work and group decision making', *ACM Computing Surveys*, 20, pp. 115–146.

Krcmar, H. and Schwabe, G. (1995) 'CATeam für den Gemeinderat. Szenarien und Visionen', in H. Reinermann (ed.), *Neubau der Verwaltung? Informationstechnische Realitäten und Visionen*, Heidelberg: Decker.

Krippendorff, K. (1980) *Content Analysis: An Introduction to Its Methodologies*, New York: Sage.

Kubicek, H., Dutton, W.H. and Williams, R. (eds) (1997) *The Social Shaping of Information Superhighways*, Frankfurt: Campus Verlag.

Kuhn, T.S. (1970) *The Structure of Scientific Revolutions*, Chicago: Chicago University Press.

Ladd, E.C. (1985) *The American Polity: The People and Their Government*, New York: Norton, as quoted in Yankelovich, D. (1991) *Coming to Public Judgement: Making Democracy Work in a Complex World*, Syracuse: Syracuse University Press.

Landers, R.K. (1988) 'Why America doesn't vote', *Editorial Research Reports*, F19, pp. 82–95.

Larsson, T. (1994) *Det svenska statsskicket*, Lund: Studentlitteratur.

Lash, S. and Urry, J. (eds) (1994) *Economies of Signs and Space*, London: Sage.

Laudon, K.C. (1977) *Communications Technology and Democratic Participation*, New York: Praeger.

Lenk, K. (1976) 'Partizipationsfördernde Technologien?', in K. Lenk (ed.), *Informationsrechte und Kommunikationspolitik*, Darmstadt: Toeche-Mittler.

Lenk, K. *et al.* (1990) *Bürgerinformationssysteme. Strategien zur Steigerung der Verwaltungstransparenz und der Partizipationschancen der Bürger*. Opladen: Westd. Verlag.

Lievesey-Howarth, R. (1997) 'Electronic governance: The risk to society', *The Australian*, 25 July, pp. 32–33.

Lippmann, W. (1960) *Public Opinion*, New York: Macmillan.

Loader, B.D. (ed.) (1997) *The Governance of Cyberspace: Politics, Technology and Global Restructuring*, London: Routledge.

Loader, B.D. (ed.) (1998) *The Cyberspace Divide: Equality, Agency and Policy in the Information Society*, London: Routledge.

Local Government Information Unit (LGIU) (1996) *A Watching Brief: A Code of Practice for CCTV*, London: LGIU.

Lyon, D. (1994) *The Electronic Eye: The Rise of the Surveillance Society*, Cambridge: Polity Press.

McChesney, R. (1997) *Corporate Media and the Threat to Democracy*, New York: Seven Stories Press.

McGrew, A. (1997) (ed.) *The Transformation of Democracy*, Cambridge: Polity Press.

McGuigan, J. (1996) *Culture and the Public Sphere*, London: Routledge.

MacKenzie, D. and Wajcman, J. (1985) *The Social Shaping of Technology: How the Refrigerator Got its Hum*, Philadelphia: Open University Press.

MacKie-Mason, J. and Varian, H. (1995) 'Pricing the internet', in B. Kahin and J. Keller (eds), *Public Access to the internet*, Cambridge, MA: MIT Press, pp. 269–314.

McLeish, H. (1998) 'Scottish CCTV Challenge Competition – 1998', *The Herald*, 28 February, p. 11.

Madaras, A. (1997, April). Personal Interview with A. Madaras, Project Manager and Producer, The Democracy Network, Center for Governmental Studies.

Malina, A. and Jankowski, N. (1998) 'Community building in Cyberspace', *Javnost/the public*, 5, 2, pp. 35–48.

Markoff, J. (1996) *Waves of Democracy: Social Movements and Political Change*, London: Sage.

Marshall, T.H. (ed.) (1973) *Class, Citizenship and Social Development*, Westport: Greenwood Press.

Martin, J. (1996) *Cybercorp: The New Business Revolution*, New York: American Management Association.

May, J. (1978) 'Defining democracy: A bid for coherence and consensus', *Political Studies*, 26, 1, pp. 1–14.

May, M. (1996) 'Surveillance: someone to watch over you', *The Daily Telegraph*, Connected, 21 May, pp. 8–9.

Mayer, I. (1997) *Debating Technologies. A Methodological Contribution to the Design and Evaluation of Participatory Policy Analysis*, Tilburg: Tilburg University Press.

Mayhew, L. (1997) *The New Public: Professional Communication and the Means of Social Influence*, Cambridge: Cambridge University Press.

Meehan, E. (1994) *Citizenship and the European Community*, London: Sage.

Meyrowitz, J. (1985) *No Sense of Place*, New York: Oxford University Press.

Michels, R. (1962) *Political Parties: A Sociological Study of the Oligarchical Tendencies of Modern Democracy*, New York: Collier.

Miller, D. on the web at http://panizzi.shef.ac.uk/community/papers.html

Miller, G. (1997) 'The impact of economics on contemporary political science', *Journal of Economic Literature*, 35, pp. 1173–1204.

Milner, E. (1997) 'Information management and its relationship to ICTs,' unpublished consultancy report.

Mitchell, W.C. and Munger, M.C. (1991) 'Economic models of interest groups: An introductory survey', *American Journal of Political Science*, 35, 2, pp. 221–232.

MORI (1996) *Disconnect Research*, London: MORI.

Musso, J., Weare, C. and Hale, M. (1998) *Using web Technology for Local Governance Reform: Good Management or Good Democracy?* Working Paper, Southern California Studies Center, University of Southern California

National Council for Civil Liberties (Liberty) (1989) *Who's Watching You? Video Surveillance in Public Places*, Briefing No. 16, London: Liberty.

National Voter Registration Act of 1993 (1994) Pub. L. No. 103–31, 107 Stat. 77 codified at 42 U.S.C. 1973 gg. *et seq.*

Naughton, E.J. (1992), 'Is cyberspace a public forum? Computer bulletin boards, free speech, and state action', *Georgetown University Law Journal*, 81, pp. 409–441.

Negroponte, N. (1995) *Being Digital*, New York: Knopf.

NetPanel (1997) available at *Digitale burger heeft weinig belangstelling voor politiek op het internet*, http://www.netpanel.nl.nieuws/pers4.html

Neuman, W.R. (1991) *The Future of the Mass Audience*, Cambridge: Cambridge University Press.

Newton, K. (1996) *Social Capital, Trust and Confidence in Advanced Democracies*, paper presented at the conference on the Erosion of Confidence in Advanced Democracies, Palais des Academies, Brussels, 7–9 November.

Niskanen, W.A. (1971) *Bureaucracy and Representative Government*, Chicago: Aldine-Atherton.

Noble, P. (1997) *Guide to the internet and Politics*, Washington, DC: C & E.

Nordilinger, E.A. (1983) *On the Autonomy of the Democratic State*, Cambridge, MA: Harvard University Press, as quoted in Barber, B. (1984) *Strong Democracy: Participatory Politics for a New Age*, Berkeley: University of California Press.

Oakerson, R. (1988) 'Reciprocity: A bottom-up view of political development', in V. Ostrum, D. Feeny and H. Picht (eds), *Rethinking Institutional Analysis and Development*, San Francisco: ICS Press.

Olsen, M. (1965) *The Logic of Collective Action*, Cambridge, MA: Harvard University Press.

Orwell, G. (1949) *Nineteen Eighty-Four*, Cutchogue, NY: Buccaneer Books.

Orwell, G. (1965) *Nineteen Eighty-Four*, London: Heinemann.

Ostrom, E. (1990) *Governing the Commons: The Evolution of Institutions for Collective Action*, New York: Cambridge University Press.

Ostrom, E. (1998) 'A behavior approach to the rational-choice theory of collective action', *American Political Science Review*, 92, 1, pp. 1–23.

Paletz, D.L. (1996) 'Advanced information technology and political communication', *Social Science Computer Review*, 14, 1, pp. 75–77.

Palfrey, T.R. and Rosenthal, H. (1988) 'Private incentives in social dilemmas', *Journal of Public Economics*, 35, 3 pp. 309–332.

Pasian, B. (1998) paper presented to the Governments on the Net '98 Conference, Ottawa, April, available at http://www.cisti.nrc.ca/forum/govnet98/speakers_e.html

Pateman, C. (1970) *Participation and Democratic Theory*, New York: Cambridge University Press.

Perritt, H.H. (1992) 'Tort liability, the First Amendment, and equal access to electronic networks', *Harvard Journal of Law and Technology*, 5, p. 65.

Perritt, H.H. (1993) 'The Congress, the courts and computer-based communication networks: Answering questions about access and control', *Villanova Law Review*, 38, pp. 319–348.

Petersson, O. (1996) *Politikens möjligheter*, Stockholm: SNS Förlag.

Petersson, O. (1998) *Svensk politik*, Stockholm: Norstedts Juridik.

Petracca, M.P. (1991) 'The rational choice approach to politics: A challenge to democratic politics', *Review of Politics*, 53, pp. 289–319.

Pinch, T. and Bijker, W. (1987) 'The social construction of facts and artifacts', in W.E. Bijker, T.P. Hughes and T. Pinch (eds), *The Social Construction of Technological Systems*, Cambridge, MA: MIT Press.

Pitkin, H.F. (1967) *The Concept of Representation*, Berkeley, CA: University of California Press.

Plant, R., Lesser, H. and Taylor-Gooby, P. (1980) *Political Philosophy and Social Welfare*, London: Routledge & Kegan Paul.

Pool, I. de Sola (1983) *Technologies of Freedom*, Cambridge, MA: Harvard University Press.

Pool, I. de Sola (1984) 'Competition and universal service: Can we get there from here?', in H.M. Shooshan (ed.), *Disconnecting Bell: The Impact of the AT&T Divestiture, New York: Pergamon*.

Putnam, R. (1993a) *Making Democracy Work*, Princeton: Princeton University Press.

Putnam, R. (1993b) 'The prosperous community: Social capital and public life,' The American Prospect, 13, pp. 35–42.

Putnam, R. (1995) 'Tuning in, tuning out: The strange disappearance of social capital in America', *PS. Political Science and Politics*, 28, 4, pp. 664–671.

Putnam, R.D. (1996) 'The strange dissapearance of civic America', *The American Prospect*, no. 24 available at http://epn.org/prospect/24/24putn.html

Rand Corporation, *Universal Access to E mail: Feasibility and Societal Implications* on the web at http://www.rand.org/publications/MR/MR650/mr650.ch7/ch7.html

Ree, J. (1984) *Proletrarian Philosophers*, Oxford: Clarendon.

Reno V. American Civil Liberties Union et al., 117 S. Ct. 2329 (1997).

Rheingold, H. (1993) *The Virtual Community*, Reading, MA: Addison-Wesley.

Richardson, J. (1994) *The Market for Political Activism: Interest Groups as a Challenge to Political Parties* (Jean Monnet Chair Papers no. 18, The Robert Schuman Centre at the European University Institute).

Robins, K. and Webster, F. (eds) (1988) *The Political Economy of Information*, Wisconsin: University of Wisconsin Press.

Rocco, E. and Warglien, M. (1995) 'Computer mediated communication and the emergence of electronic opportunism. Working paper RCC 13659. Venice, Italy: Universita Degli Studi di Venezia, as cited in F. Ostrom (1998) 'A behavior approach to the rational-choice theory of collective action, *American Political Science Review*, 92, 1, pp. 1–23.

Rosell. S.A., et al. (1995) *Changing Maps*, Ottawa: Carleton University Press.

Ross, D. and Hood, J. (1998) 'Closed circuit television (CCTV) – the Easterhouse case study', in L. Montaheiro, et al. (eds), *Public and Private Sector Partnerships: Fostering Enterprise*, Sheffield: Sheffield Hallam University Press.

Ryan, A. (1995) *John Dewey*, New York, W.W. Norton.

Sackman, H. and Nie, N. (eds) (1970) *The Information Utility and Social Choice*, Montvale, NJ: AFIPS Press.

Sackman, H. and Boehm, B. (eds) (1972) *Planning Community Information Utilities*, Montvale, NJ: AFIPS Press.

Sally, D. (1995) 'Conversation and cooperation in social dilemmas: A meta-analysis of experiments from 1958 to 1992', *Rationality and Society*, 7, 1, pp. 58–92.

Schalken, C.A.T. (1998) 'Internet as a new public sphere for democracy?', in I.Th.M. Snellen and W.B.H.J. van de Donk (eds), *Public Administration in an Information Age: A Handbook*, Amsterdam: IOS Press.

Schalken, C.A.T. and Tops, P.W. (1995) 'Democracy and virtual communities. An empirical exploration of the Amsterdam digital city', in W.B.H.J. van de Donk, *et al.*, *Orwell in Athens: A Perspective on Informatization and Democracy*, Amsterdam: IOS Press.

Schalken, K. (1997) *Internet as a New Public Sphere for Politics and Democracy*, paper presented at Images of Politics Conference, Amsterdam October 23–25.

Schiller, H. (1996) *Information Inequality: The Deepening Social Crisis in America*, London: Routledge.

Schneider, S. (1996) 'Creating a democratic public sphere through political discussion', *Social Science Computer Review*, 14, pp. 373–393.

Schudson, M. (1997) 'Why conversation is not the soul of democracy', *Critical Studies in Mass Communication*, 14, pp. 297–309.

Schwabe, G. (1994) *Computerunterstützte Sitzungen. Stuttgart* (Arbeitspapiere des Lehrstuhls für Wirtschaftsinformatik der Universität Hohenheim Nr. 59).

Schwartz, E. (1996) *Netactivism: How Citizens Use the internet*, Cambridge, MA: O'Reilly.

Scientific and Technological Options Assessment Unit (STOA) (1998) *An Appraisal of Technologies of Political Control (Working Document)*, European Parliament, Directorate General for Research, The STOA Programme, Luxembourg: European Parliament.

Sclove, R.E. (1992) 'The nuts and bolts of democracy: Democratic theory and technical design', in L. Winner (ed.), *Democracy in a Technological Society*, London: Kluwer Academic.

Sclove, R.E. (1995) *Democracy and Technology*, New York: Guildford Press.

Scott, J. (1991) *Social Network Analysis*, London: Sage.

The Scottish Council for Civil Liberties (SCCL) (1994) *Civil Liberties and Video Cameras*, Briefing No. 2, Glasgow: SCCL.

Scottish Office (1996a) *Closed Circuit Television Challenge Competition 1996–97: Successful Applications*, Scottish Office: Crime Prevention Unit.

Scottish Office (1996b) *CCTV in Scotland: A Framework for Action*, Scotland: HMSO.

Scottish Office (1997) *Closed Circuit Television Challenge Competition 1997–98: Applications Recommended for Approval*, Scottish Office: Crime Prevention Unit.

Scottish Office (1998) *CCTV Challenge Competition 1998–9: Successful Applications*, Scottish Office: Crime Prevention Unit.

Sell, J. and Wilson, R. (1991) 'Levels of information and contributions to public goods', *Social Forces*, 70, 1, pp. 107–124.

Sell, J. and Wilson, R. (1992) 'Liar, liar, pants on fire: Cheap talk and signalling in repeated public goods settings,' Working paper, Houston, TX: Rice University, Department of Political Science, as cited in E. Ostrom (1998) 'A behavior approach to the rational-choice theory of collective action', *American Political Science Review*, 92, 1, pp. 1–23.

Shapiro, J. (1994) 'Three ways to be a democrat', *Political Theory*, 22, pp. 124–151.

Sheekey, A. (1997) *Education and Telecommunications: Critical Issues and Resources*, Boston: Information Gatekeeper.

Shenk, D. (1997) *Data Smog: Surviving the Information Glut*, New York: HarperCollins.

Short, E. and Ditton, J. (1995) 'Does CCTV affect crime?', *CCTV Today*, 2, 2, pp. 10–12.

Sjölin, M. (1994) 'Massmedier och opinionsbildning', in A. Sannerstedt and M. Jerneck (eds), *Den moderna demokratins problem*, Lund: Studentlitteratur.

Slaton, C.D. (1992) *Televote: Expanding Citizen Participation in the Quantum Age*, New York: Praeger.

Smith, C. (1997) *Political Parties in the Information Age: From 'Mass Party' to Leadership Organisation*, paper presented to the XIth meeting of the Permanent Study Group on Informatization in Public Administration. European Group of Public Administration Annual Conference, Leuven, 9–13 September.

Smith, M. (1996) 'Alone at the polls: a national embarrassment', *Social Polity*, 27, pp. 4–9.

Snoddy, R. (1997), 'Time Warner to end interactive service', *Financial Times*, 2 May.

Southern, A. (1997) 'Re-booting the local economy', *Local Economy: The Journal of the Local Economy Policy Unit*, 12, 1, pp. 8–25.

Southwell, P.L. (1986) 'Alienation and nonvoting in the United States: Crucial interactive effects among independent variables', *Journal of Political and Military Sociology*, 14, 2, pp. 249–261.

Spears, R. and Lea, M. (1994) 'Panacea or panopticon? The hidden power in computer-mediated communication', *Communication Research*, 21, pp. 427–459.

Sproull, L. and Faraj, S. (1995) 'Atheism, sex, and databases: The net as a social technology', in B. Kahin and J. Keller (eds), *Public Access to the internet*, Cambridge, MA: MIT Press, pp. 62–81.

Steinmüller, W. (1993) *Informationstechnologie und Gesellschaft. Einführung in die angewandte Informatik*, Darmstadt: Wiss. Buchges.

Stevens, J.B. (1993) *The Economics of Collective Choice*, Boulder, CO: Westview.

Stigler, G. (1971) 'The theory of economic regulation', *The Bell Journal of Economics and Management Science*, 2, 1, pp. 98–129.

Stodder, M. (1997, March). Personal interview with M. Stodder, Project Director, The Democracy Network, Center for Governmental Studies.

Stone, P.J., Dunphy, D.C., Smith, M.S. and Ogilvie, D.M. (1966) *The General Inquirer: A Computer Approach to Content Analysis*, Cambridge, MA: MIT Press.

Strathclyde Police Media and Information Services (1996) *CityWatch: The Story So Far*, press release, 28 May, Glasgow: Strathclyde Police Force.

Stratton Oakmont, Inc. v. Prodigy Services Co., 23 Media L. Rep. 1794 (1995).

Street, H. (1972) *Freedom. The Individual and The Law*, 3rd edition, London: Penguin.

Szretter 'Social capital, the economy and the Third Way', Nexus paper on the web at http://www.netnexus.org/3wayecon/library/socialcap.htm

Taviss, M.L. (1992). 'Dueling forums: The public forum doctrine's failure to protect the electronic forum', *University of Cincinatti Law Review*, 60, pp. 757–795.

Taylor, M. and Saarinen, E. (1994) *Imagologies: Media Philosophy*, New York: Routledge.

Taylor, R. (1997) 'Chattering against Mr Blair', *The Spectator*, 19 April, p. 11.

Thompson, B. and Aikens, G.S. (1998) 'If Jefferson had had e-mail', *The New Statesman*, 20 February, p. 22.

Thompson, G. (1993) 'Network coordination', in R. Maidment and G. Thompson (eds), *Managing the United Kingdom*, London: Sage.

Thompson, J. (1995) *Media and Modernity*, Oxford: Polity Press.

Tops, P. and Depla, P. (1997) *Dutch Political Parties in the Digital Era: The Technological Challenge*, paper presented at Images of Politics Conference, Amsterdam, 23–25 October.

UK Communities Online on the web at http://www.communities.org.uk

UK National Working Party on Social Inclusion (1997) The Net Result: Report of the UK National Working Party on Social Inclusion on the web at http://www.uk.ibm.com/community/uk117.html

US Telecom Reform Bill 1996.

Verba, S., Schlozman, Lehman, K. and Brady, H.E. (1995) *Voice and Equality: Civic Voluntarism in American Politics*, Cambridge, MA: MIT Press.

Vickers, G. (1995) *The Art of Judgement: A Study of Policy Making*, Advances in Public Administration Series, London: Sage.

Ward, M. (1996) 'The effect of the internet on political institutions', *Industrial and Corporate Change*, 5, 4, pp. 1127–1142.

Weare, C., Musso, J.A. and Hale, M. (1999) 'Electronic democracy and the diffusion of municipal web pages in California,' *Administration and Society*.

Weber, R.P. (1990) *Basic Content Analysis*, Newbury Park: Sage.

Webster, C.W.R. (1996) 'Closed circuit television and governance: The eve of a surveillance age', *Information Infrastructure and Policy*, 5, 4, pp. 253–263.

Webster, C.W.R. (1998) 'Changing relationships between citizens and the state: the case of closed circuit television surveillance cameras', in I.Th.M. Snellen and W.B.H.J. van de Donk, *Public Administration in an Information Age: A Handbook*. Informatization Developments and the Public Sector Series, no. 6. Amsterdam: IOS Press.

Webster, C.W.R. (1999) 'Relegitimating the democratic polity: The closed circuit television revolution in the UK', in I. Horrocks, J. Hoff and P. Tops, *Democratic Governance and New Technology: Technologically Mediated Innovations in Political Practice in Western Europe*, London: Routledge.

Webster, F. (1996) *Theories of the Information Society*, London: Routledge.

Wellman, B. and Berkowitz, S.D. (1988) *Social Structures*, Cambridge: Cambridge University Press.

Westen, T. (1997, January), Personal interview with T. Westen, President, Center for Governmental Studies.

Westen, T. and Givens, B. (1989) *The California Channel: A New Public Affairs Television Network for the State*, Los Angeles, CA: Center for Governmental Studies.

Westerbrook, R. (1991) *John Dewey and American Democracy*, New York: Cornell University Press.

Wilhelm, A. (1997) 'A resource model of computer-mediated political life', *Policy Studies Journal*, 25, pp. 519–534.

Wilkinson, H. and Mulgan, G. (1995) *Freedom's Children: Work Relationships and Politics for 18–34 Year Olds in Britain Today*, London: DEMOS.

Williams, F. (1982) *The Communications Revolution*, Beverly Hills: Sage.

Williams, R. and Edge, D. (1996), 'The social shaping of technology', in W.H. Dutton (ed.), *Information and Communication Technologies: Visions and Realities*, Oxford: Oxford University Press.

Winner, L. (1986) *The Whale and the Reactor: A Search for Limits in an Age of High Technology*, Chicago: University of Chicago Press.

Winner, L. (ed.) (1992) *Democracy in a Technological Society*, London: Kluwer Academic Publishers.

Wright, T. (1994) *Citizens and Subjects*, London: Routledge.

Yankelovich, D. (1991) *Coming to Public Judgement: Making Democracy Work in a Complex World*, Syracuse: Syracuse University Press.

Yzerbyt, V., Leyens, J.-P. and Bellour, F. (1995) 'The ingroup overexclusion effect: Identity concerns in discussion about group membership', *European Journal of Social Psychology*, 25, pp. 239–250.

Index